613.25 QUI

MAR      2014

Quince, Dolvett

The 3-1-2-1 diet : eat and
cheat your way to weight
loss-- up to 10 pounds in
21 days

# THE
# 3-1-2-1
# DIET

# Dolvett Quince

with Maggie Greenwood-Robinson

# THE 3-1-2-1 DIET

EAT *AND* CHEAT YOUR WAY
TO WEIGHT LOSS—UP TO
10 POUNDS IN 21 DAYS

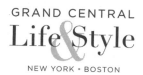

GRAND CENTRAL
Life & Style

NEW YORK • BOSTON

Grand Central Life & Style
Hachette Book Group
237 Park Avenue
New York, NY 10017
www.GrandCentralLifeandStyle.com

Printed in the United States of America

RRD-C

First Edition: November 2013

10 9 8 7 6 5 4 3

Grand Central Life & Style is an imprint of Grand Central Publishing.

The Grand Central Life & Style name and logo are trademarks of Hachette Book Group, Inc.

All other trademarks used in this book are the property of their respective owners.

The Hachette Speakers Bureau provides a wide range of authors for speaking events. To find out more, go to www.HachetteSpeakersBureau.com or call (866) 376-6591.

The publisher is not responsible for websites (or their content) that are not owned by the publisher.

Library of Congress Cataloging-in-Publication Data

Quince, Dolvett.
The 3-1-2-1 diet : eat and cheat your way to weight loss—up to 10 pounds in 21 days / Dolvett Quince.—First edition.
ISBN 978-1-4555-7672-2 (hardback)—ISBN 978-1-4555-7671-5 (ebook)
1. Weight loss—Popular works. 2. Exercise—Popular works. 3. Reducing diets—Popular works. I. Title. II. Title: Three-one-two-one diet.
RM222.2.Q85 2014
613.2'5—dc23                    2013030418

*First, I dedicate this book to you, and for you, in order to show you that all things are possible. Believe in yourself, trust in God and watch your dreams unfold!!*

*Second, I dedicate this book to my son, Isiah. My prayer for you is to be open.*

*Open your eyes to see beyond what's in front of you. Open your ears to hear music all the time. Most of all, open your heart…period.*

# ACKNOWLEDGMENTS

I'm so excited about acknowledging the following people (my power team!) for their work, help, and contributions to this book: Lee Kernis, Jaime Roberts, Don Epstein, Kelly Mendelsohn, Maggie Greenwood-Robinson, Diana Baroni, and Amanda Englander. Thank you for helping me with a book that I hope will help many people live healthier, more balanced, and happier lives.

# CONTENTS

## PART FOUR:  *More Tools from My Toolbox*

# INTRODUCTION

## A Real Diet for Real Life

This is going to be the best, simplest diet you've ever been on. I know, because it gives you three things that people have been telling me they want ever since I became a personal trainer more than twenty years ago.

The first thing is a diet that really works, in real life, for real people. Not some trendy, drink-soup-all-day or snack-on-celery-until-you-turn-green diet that's hard to start and hard to stay on. No, what you and everyone else want is a diet that takes off pounds steadily and that you can follow without feeling hungry or deprived—an easy-to-do diet that you can actually stick to. I get that. Did you know, for example, that most women give up diets after 5 weeks, 2 days, and 43 minutes? Yep. That's what the current research says. Trust me, you won't be one of those statistics on this diet.

The second thing people want is a diet that drops weight pretty fast—no plateaus, no slowdowns, just results they can see on the scale and in the mirror. And there's nothing wrong with that. Research now shows that when people experience accelerated results, they tend to be more motivated to stay on their diets and they're more likely to keep the weight off.

And most important, the third thing people kept telling me they want can be summed up in three words: ability to cheat. You read that right. You want a diet you can cheat on and still lose weight. A diet with really good strategies to let you eat ice cream, pizza, macaroni and cheese—whatever you want—but without beating yourself up and vowing never to do it again. On this diet, you can have anything your heart desires, 2 days a week, as long as moderation and portion control are your MOs. You won't feel deprived because you'll be allowing yourself your favorite foods a few times a week.

The 3-1-2-1 Diet delivers all three things you and many others want.

As for the cheating part, I'll bet most of you don't believe that you can cheat a little and lose a lot of weight. You think you've got to starve yourself down to a thinner size.

I'll prove that the opposite is true.

Or maybe you think you've got to spend exhausting hours in the gym, sweating yourself silly, every day, to burn off fat.

Again, not true.

If you continue to believe that you have to deprive yourself of food or that you have to work out until you drop, then you will miss out on the transformation of a lifetime.

I won't let that happen.

And that's where this book comes in—*The 3-1-2-1 Diet*. For years I've been giving this diet to my clients, and it's been highly successful. It involves 3 days of clean eating, followed by 1 cheat day, then 2 days of clean eating, and 1 more cheat day. You stick to that pattern of eating, week after week, and the pounds will melt off. I won't be forcing you to do anything drastic, like superstrict dieting or meal-planning pyramids or fat-gram counting. I tried all that early in my career, and my clients rebelled—and so did their bodies, by clinging to fat rather than releasing it. Instead of depriving you and denying you foods, I'm giving you permission to eat virtually any food you want. Granted, I'll give it to you in doses and in moderation. But I won't take away from your lifestyle. I'll enhance your lifestyle and show you how to form new, realistic habits that will stay with you for a lifetime. I take a lot of pride in getting real results for real people, and that's what you'll get on this diet. In fact, you can lose up to 10 pounds in just 21 days! You'll keep losing until you reach your goal weight—and I'll show you how to finally keep it off forever.

The 3-1-2-1 Diet works by manipulating your body's natural tendency to slow its metabolic rate in response to severe calorie restriction. It takes a new approach to getting lean, one scientifically based on changing up food and calories to tap into your body's potential to burn fat. You'll lose weight fast and you won't plateau. While unconventional, my diet will give you greater amounts of muscle and less fat than practically anything you've ever tried.

On my 3-1-2-1 Diet, you'll discover how to:

■  Enjoy a flexible plan that will fit your food preferences and your lifestyle.
■  "Cheat" your way to a faster metabolism and leaner body.

- Lose weight—up to 10 pounds during the first 21 days—beginning the very first day, and keep losing weight steadily, right down to your goal.
- Prepare delicious, easy-to-fix meals with the help of my meal plans and recipes that help you burn fat and improve your health.
- Feel satisfied—no hunger pangs or cravings.
- Get supertoned and fit by following a simple 48-minute workout that combines cardio and body-shaping moves.

So let me ask you: Are you ready for your transformation? Are you ready to learn a new way of living that will change your body, your attitude, and your life? In just 21 days you will look and feel better and be on your way to an all-new you.

# TRUST THE JOURNEY

Since we'll be working together on every page of this book, let me tell you about who I am and how I got involved in health and fitness. I live by the principles in this plan and I keep myself motivated—that's how I get results. As you probably know, I have been one of the trainers on NBC's *The Biggest Loser* for 4 seasons. I'm also a personal trainer and a motivational speaker. But what you may not know is that getting to this point in my life has definitely been a journey—and not an easy one.

On season 13 of *The Biggest Loser*, a contestant named Jeremy started training with me. He was in a bad mental funk because he was getting close to leaving the ranch. I wanted to encourage him, you know, to keep on keeping on.

"Trust the journey," I told him. "You are a fighter. Fighters don't quit. Fighters don't whine or complain. They do the work...so do the work. Don't fall in love with the end goal. Fall in love with the journey and make it your life."

Think about what that means. To me, it means success is moving forward, finding out what works and what doesn't, and challenging yourself to be your best. It's the way we travel on that journey, at least to me, that's most important. People who are really successful enjoy the journey as much as the destination.

This is a lesson I have been learning all my life, because I was not always the Dolvett Quince you see today. As a child, I was told that I would never amount to anything and that I wouldn't succeed in life.

I grew up in Stamford, Connecticut, in a poor home without a father. My mother was barely out of her teens when she gave birth to me, the third of four kids. My two brothers, Andrew (the oldest) and Joey (the youngest), one sister, Lavonne, and I were caught in a web of poverty and neglect. We lived in a deteriorating apartment in the projects, where rats crawled across our feet. We were left by ourselves all day long, while my mother spent many hours out searching for my father, to see whom he was messing with.

Our neighbors started complaining, and before long, Social Services intervened. One day, they swept in and took us. My mom walked in after them, screaming, "Where are you taking my babies?" As I was being dragged off, I dropped my teddy bear, whose name was Blue, and he fell under a table. I stretched out my arms, but I couldn't get to him. He was being left behind, and I felt a part of me was being left behind too. My life was different after that, and I was only four years old.

My brother Joey, who was one at the time, and I were sent to a stranger's home, a foster home. My older brother and sister went to a different foster home. I thought I would never see them again.

My aunt Joan saw the heartbreak of us being yanked from our mother and separated from each other. She fought hard with Social Services to get us placed in a foster home together. After 4 weeks, she was successful. The four of us were sent to a foster home in the suburbs of Bridgeport, a far cry from the projects where we used to live. Our foster parents seemed wealthy, and they had a huge home, where they took in foster kids. There were about fifteen other children living there when we moved in.

Oddly, though, the foster kids there seemed to be shuttled in and out constantly. One week, three would leave; another week, five were gone. I'd wake up every morning and tell my sister, "We're going next." I was scared.

Then one day we woke up, and all the foster children were gone except us. For 6 months, it was just the four of us, no other kids.

My foster parents came to us and said, "We want to know if you four would like to be with us forever. We have been praying about this, and we want to adopt you."

I was listening to their words, but it felt like they were asking, "Do you want a million dollars?"

And so we were adopted, all four of us. We had gone from the projects to a palace.

It was, on the surface, a happy, privileged family tableau. But we lived a deeply unhappy childhood under that roof.

You see, our adoptive parents were old school Jamaican; they seemed to believe that if you spare the rod, you spoil the child. So my dad would twist a switch from a tree or yank an electrical cord from the wall and whip us on the butt or legs or across the knuckles. Sometimes he used his fist. And sometimes we'd bleed or be left with welts on our legs. He felt a need to control us that way, hoping to prevent us from acting up or getting out of place, to beat the badness out of us. I remember feeling so helpless.

My mom made us wear the same clothes to school Monday through Friday, a hold-over from the Jamaican custom of students wearing uniforms to school. I'd argue with her, "Mom, all the kids wear different clothes. They're laughing at us." She didn't care; that was her rule.

And then there were the put-downs. We were constantly reminded that we weren't theirs, that if we didn't like the rules, we could leave.

I was the darkest-skinned one of the four; my siblings were fair. I was called "Blackie Bo," and it stung.

My father said to me one time, "Andrew is the oldest. Lavonne is my only girl, and Joey is the baby. What do you think that means you are to me? Nothing."

Our self-esteem suffered as a result of that upbringing, and they taught us to hate ourselves.

But I found myself fighting back, harshly sometimes, while my siblings shrank from the conflict. Our parents' stinging words and ways stuck with them for life. Even today my sister and brothers struggle with their insecurities that stem from this upbringing.

I often wonder what made me different. After all, we grew up in the same house and experienced the same pain, the doubt, and the low self-esteem. If any of us should have been screwed up, it should have been me, since I had suffered the most emotional abuse.

But I had grit. I had a voice. It empowered me. I learned early on that pain is going to come to you, and people aren't going to like you, but *you* need to learn to never stop liking you. Unlike my brothers and sister, I let the emotional abuse go, and I practiced letting it go. I kept working on making my spirit strong, just like you'd develop a muscle to be strong. I believe that it is that inner strength that ultimately empowered me to empower other people, because I know what it is like to doubt yourself. You start to believe in your "I can'ts." "I can't lose weight. I can't do those squats. I can't get to any of my goals. I can't ever be anyone." And on and on.

All the time I was living with my adoptive parents, I wanted to get away. I just kept thinking that this was some horrible transition, a nasty time. I stayed there and toughed it out, until one day, at age thirteen, I *did* leave. My friend's mom let me stay with them for about six months. Then I went back, and things were worse. Gradually, my siblings left, one by one. They just couldn't take it anymore. None of us felt wanted.

There were times I'd ask God, "What are you thinking? You took me from one terrible situation and put me in another."

The book of Jeremiah says, " 'For I know the plans I have for you,' declares the Lord, 'plans to prosper you and not to harm you, plans to give you hope and a future.' "

I clung to the hope expressed in that scripture and began to see some positives. One was that God had surrounded me with people I looked up to, namely, a man named Mr. Adams, who was a neighbor, a lawyer, an elder in our church, and a friend of my parents. Well dressed and well spoken, he had four boys and a beautiful wife. But my admiration for this extraordinary man goes beyond just his successful lifestyle. He was kind, loving, and strong. He counseled people in the church community, including my parents. I looked up to him, and I wanted to be like him. And I knew in my heart it was possible.

At fourteen years old, I walked into a gym one day. I was petrified. But as I looked around the room, the air heavy with the smell of sweat, my fears soon left me. I began to create a vision of myself going from scrawny to strong. I walked up to a trainer and told him I wanted to learn how to lift weights and build some muscle. He took one look at me and said, "Okay, kid, whatever. Let's work on your legs first and go from there."

I was excited.

I kept at it. One day, I caught my reflection in a car window, and I looked huge and ripped. My string-bean body had responded quickly to the rigors of weight training. It changed my life, and I got hooked.

My passion for fitness grew. To make some money, I started working at the front desk of a local YMCA. A co-worker approached me one day and said, "You are good with people. You have a good physique. Have you thought about being a trainer?"

The idea took hold in my head and heart—it made sense—so I got certified and became a trainer at the local YMCA. It was crazy. I had gone to the gym in search of just muscles but then found a calling—to become a personal trainer. I realized that I could take all of that energy and passion I had for fitness and help others discover the benefits of exercise and a healthy diet. Becoming a personal trainer was the best thing that ever happened to me. I was twenty-two years old.

Before long, I was developing programs for sedentary moms and working with pudgy middle-aged men. I'll never forget one of my earliest clients, Erica, who was 60 pounds overweight and wanted to shape up for her wedding. I started training her. We talked about nutrition and what she should eat. Before long, she started dropping weight like crazy. A week before her wedding, Erica had achieved her goal. She looked amazing—shapely, defined—gorgeous, really. She came to me in tears and handed me a Gap gift card. This was the very first time I had received a gift as a trainer, and I was so moved. It was a small gift but it touched my heart in a big way. Then she said, "Because of you, I'm going to have the best day of my life." I knew in that moment I was doing what I was destined to do.

I loved being a personal trainer. I kept my work personal, listening to my clients, connecting with them, and helping them navigate through the emotional pain that was so often responsible for the shape they were in. I felt a responsibility for helping people, inside and out.

Every day was like school for me. I discovered that diet and exercise were two of the toughest areas of a person's life to change—and I was being asked to change both. I picked everyone's brains about diet, nutrition, working out, health, and more. I was thirsty and drank deeply from the well of knowledge and experience of those around me.

As a personal trainer, I began to meet all kinds of interesting people, from all walks of life, and things were going along very well. I was living in Atlanta, Georgia, at the time, and working at a large gym. I noticed a guy who worked out there, Bert Weiss. He was doing everything wrong and not making much progress. His potential was going to waste, so I kept badgering him to hire me as his trainer, or at least work out with me. He declined, but I persisted. After 2 months, he relented and did a workout with me. Five minutes into the workout, he realized he needed to work out faster, harder, and just differently altogether. He became one of my clients and, instantly, one of my best friends. To this day, we speak every day. We have a lot in common: Not only are we both from broken homes, but we also both have a deep sense of family, we're both music lovers, and we have many other areas of commonality as well.

A few months after we started training together, I found out that he was the number one radio talk-show host in Atlanta—the "Bert" from *The Bert Show.* He called me up one day and asked me to come on his show and talk about fitness. Naturally, I agreed to do it, although I was as nervous as— (He advised me to clean up my act a bit, because back then I did curse a lot!)

Long story short, I started appearing on his radio show as a regular. I told listeners that I could transform Bert's body in 3 months. At the time, he was still puffy. By the end of 3 months, he had completely chiseled his physique. Local magazines and newspapers were picturing his before-and-after transformation.

All that publicity gave my personal training business a huge boost. I was getting sixty new clients a week, which was great, except that I couldn't keep up with the demand. I ended up hiring trainers to work for me, using my workout methods. At night, after training clients all day, I'd train my trainers in how to truly transform physiques. Essentially, I created a business within a business.

I approached people in my industry, asking them about how to open a gym and trying to get advice from them. They mostly laughed at me and told me I was fine where I was. But I wanted to do more. In 2003, I had made enough money to open my own personal training studio, Body Sculptor. Those same people who laughed at me leaned on me for advice and asked me how I did it.

I worked hard and built the studio into one of Atlanta's premiere health and fitness centers. A friend advised me that I needed to create my signature workout, so I invented Pure Energy, a high-intensity circuit-training class with a live DJ. It was once voted Best Workout in the Southeast.

I was pumped. For those on the go or unable to get to the gym, I created the DVD *Me and My Chair: The No Excuses Workout*, comprised of two low-impact, high-intensity 30-minute workouts that help you tone up and slim down using only a household chair.

I eventually hired a manager and a publicist. The publicist helped introduce me to more local celebrities, who became our clients. One thing led to another, and I started training a lot of nationally and internationally known celebrities. These were exciting times.

But I never lost sight of my motto: "Changing lives one rep at a time." I've always taken a lot of pride in what I do, and I pay a lot of attention to detail. I'm very involved with the development of my clients, and I'm not distracted. When someone hires me, I take them from where they are to where they should be. I don't look at myself as just a trainer; I consider myself a transformer.

These days, there are two questions I get asked the most: Are you single? (Answer: Yes.) And how did you get to be on *The Biggest Loser*?

The answer to that second question is a little more involved. Several years ago, the show was looking for a new trainer. Somehow, my name surfaced in the producer's office, so it was the show that came looking for me, not the other way around. I believe that many factors led me organically down that road, including building my career and starting to train celebrities, as well as having a private training studio in Atlanta.

Off I went to Los Angeles for an audition, which went well. It wasn't too difficult. *The Biggest Loser* crew taped an episode with me, at a hotel gym, where I trained two former contestants and two other people who hadn't done the show before. There were twenty-five trainers the first go-round. That number got scaled down, and I made it to the last three, but the producers chose someone else, so I returned to Atlanta and kept working. It was no big deal; I was so thankful even to be considered.

The show called me back 3 months later. Would I like another audition? I couldn't pack my bags fast enough. Instead of twenty-five trainers, I was the only one auditioning, and rather than a hotel gym, I was auditioning at *The Biggest Loser* Ranch, so the whole vibe felt different the second go-round. I was more confident, and they were more confident in me. And it was a good fit. Timing was everything. The rest is history, as they say. I got hired.

The experience has been a great affirmation of my calling. It's a great feeling to be a part of *The Biggest Loser* family and alumni. But I always say, stay hungry, but stay humble. At the end of the day, I just believe in hard work, wherever you are. And if you combine hard work with passion and really love what you do, good things will come back to you. So far in my own life, I think that because I gave back as much as I did, I got back as much as I did.

With this book, you're getting the real Dolvett, with a real program designed so that you can feel like I am with you every day, like I am with my *Biggest Loser* team, acting as your own personal nutrition coach and trainer. I'll shoot straight with you and tell you exactly what you need to be doing—and why. I'll give you affirmations, tips, a body-sculpting workout, and advice—everything I can think of to help you succeed. I'll be there every day to make you believe in yourself and help you be the best you can be and stay consistent in your pursuit.

If you want to lose weight and burn fat, all you have to do is follow my meal-by-meal, day-by-day guidelines and my 48-minute exercise program for the next 3 weeks and beyond. I'm not saying it will be easy. It won't. Nothing worthwhile in life really ever comes easy. But I'll be here to help you adopt a whole new lifestyle that involves a great diet, stepped-up physical activity, and a new attitude toward yourself that can enhance—and maybe even save—your life.

Along the way, there will be a lot of people who tell you that you can't do it, but don't listen to them. There are so many people in front of you who have gone down this path before you and have succeeded big-time. So don't ever, ever, *ever* give up on your dreams. Make them a reality through your words, deeds, and actions.

You are about to get some amazing results, and a few weeks from now, you'll like what you see in the mirror—you really will.

So once again, let me ask you: Are you ready for your transformation?

# THE
# 3-1-2-1
# DIET

# Part One

## 3-1-2-1—Go!

# 1 How Bad Do You Want It?

I recently read a scary statistic: By 2017, 85 percent of Americans will be very, very heavy—obese, really. That's not too far away. I fear the bad habits, the poor choices, the lack of motivation, and the non-active lifestyles that are leading people in that direction. I don't want to sound alarmist, but the truth is, people are in big trouble. You might even be one of them, and that's why you bought this book.

This is not overblown information, nor is it based on false info. This is real. This is serious. This is a big wake-up call; it's something we need to deal with before it hurts or kills us. This, folks, is our growing weight problem.

Now, you may not be obese—you may not need to lose 50, 30, or even 20 pounds—but still, I'm sure you'll agree with me: It's great to look good and be in shape. What we need to understand, though, is that excess weight isn't just a cosmetic problem; it can be a health hazard—a serious one. Controlling your weight is definitely about looking fine, but it's also about how well—and in many cases how long—you will live.

There are plenty of diets and programs out there to help, but it's likely that nothing has worked for you. Maybe you lost weight—and then gained it back. Maybe you just weren't ready to make the commitment to a healthier lifestyle. Whatever the problem, something has to change. You need to drop the weight and get healthy *once and for all*.

Enough about the bad news. The good news is that no one has to be overweight and sick. We can stop the scary side effects of obesity right now by gearing up in a positive way. In order to do that, I have a solution—a plan I've developed that has succeeded for everyone I've worked with, because it's realistic and fits into anyone's lifestyle: the 3-1-2-1 Diet. It has worked for many and it will work for you. By the way, I don't expect anyone to do anything that I don't personally do. This plan is what I live by. It's how I eat and exercise every week. And I have a big responsibility to help you do it too. I just hope you want it bad enough!

## EAT AND CHEAT

The *3* and the *2* parts of this plan are the days you're going to eat clean and healthy. The *1* part is when you get to cheat on the diet.

*Cheat? Dolvett, are you kidding me?*

No, I'm not kidding you. Practically every diet that was ever developed involves deprivation. Banned foods. Whole food groups kicked out. Illegal foods. Bad foods. Don't eat this and don't eat that. You know the drill. Although I hate the cliché, on my program, you can have your cake and eat it too.

## A HISTORY LESSON

When you go on typical diets, you lose body fat, but you also lose muscle. That's not cool, since muscle is your body's main fat-burning tissue. So after a typical deprivation-type diet, you might weigh less, but you'll have a higher percentage of fat on your body than before because of the muscle you lost. Even worse, once you return to a normal eating pattern, you're more likely to pack away extra calories as fat. The reason is that your body, in response to the decrease in calories, slows its metabolism to hold on to fat. In other words, your body doesn't think it's being fed enough, so it stores fat as if there were a famine.

When we were cave people, foraging for berries in the wild and slaying mammoths for dinner, this fat-storing factor was important for survival. The fat we stored was used for energy when food was scarce. And those who could store the most fat had an evolutionary advantage. While this was great for cave people, it sucks if you're trying to look good in a bathing suit.

How times have changed! Food is not scarce; there's a fast-food joint on every street corner. And fat people do not have an evolutionary advantage. They tend to die young, and they usually die from obesity-related diseases like heart attacks, diabetes, strokes, and even cancer.

The 3-1-2-1 Diet is not your typical diet. You won't lose muscle and you won't hold on to any fat. Keep reading, and I'll explain why.

## ON AGAIN, OFF AGAIN: IGNITE THE FAT BURN

If you've ever lifted weights or done any sort of strength training, you know how changing your routine from time to time shocks your body into getting tighter and fitter. Well, intermittent changes in your caloric intake do the same thing. On your clean days, you'll be eating fewer calories; on your cheat days, you'll be eating more calories. Those caloric ups and downs have a couple of big benefits: They trick your body into believing it has a lot of available food (which means no hoarding of fat), and they boost your metabolism, the body's food-to-fuel process, to burn fat while maintaining as much lean, sexy muscle as humanly possible. In fact, your metabolism is kept completely off balance because it's not allowed to adapt to any set level of food consumption, so it just keeps running and burning fat.

The basic weekly process is to eat clean for 3 days, cheat for 1 day, eat clean for 2 days, and cheat the next day. Obviously, the clean days will have you eating fewer calories, and the cheat days will provide slightly more calories. (See page 72 in Chapter 4 for a specific day-by-day eating guide.)

## THE C-WORD: CALORIES

According to a survey I read, more than two-thirds of our population has no clue how many calories they should eat in a day to lose weight or keep it off. And most people are eating way too many calories each day. To my way of thinking, we're in danger of becoming "calorie comatose." And that, friends, is adding to—excuse the pun—our weight problem.

So wake up. Calorie counting is *not* out of style. After decades of weight-control schemes that claim to count everything but calories, we now know what really counts: calories! We count calories on *The Biggest Loser*, and you will count them on this diet, to some extent.

In fact, diets you've been on in the past, like low-carb or low-fat diets, points-based plans, or food exchanges, are all just different ways of counting calories. And when they didn't work, it was probably because you didn't really cut down on your calories. I remember a time when low-fat diets were all the rage, and lots of fat-free foods hit the market, but dieters got fat anyway because they were unaware of all the sugar calories they were packing away by eating those fat-free foods.

Okay, for some perspective, here's a little Calories 101. A calorie is simply a type of measurement, like minutes or miles. But instead of measuring time or length, you measure the energy value of a particular portion of food. A big slab of cheesecake may have 500 calories, enough energy to get you through an intense hourlong aerobics class. But if you don't go to that class, or its equivalent, your body will store those unused calories as fat.

On your clean days, calorie counting is pretty easy, because I've done it for you through portion control on your plate. On those 2 days a week when you get to cheat, I will ask you to keep a real close eye on your calories. Women need to eat around 1,500 calories, men around 1,800. Now, before you get too excited about cheating, understand that I'm not talking about a diet free-for-all. I once had a client come into my training studio with an entire box of fresh-baked chocolate chip cookies. She was devouring them in front of me right before her workout. That is *not* the way to cheat!

## THE BIG THREE

You'll be eating the right amounts of fat, protein, carbs, and fiber for weight loss throughout this program. The diet is generally low in fat, and that's good because fat contributes more calories per gram than any other nutrient (9 calories per fat gram compared to 4 each for carbohydrates and proteins). To get lean, a great place to begin cutting calories is with your fat intake. On the 3-1-2-1 Diet, I treat fat as a condiment, like mustard or horseradish—something you use sparingly for a little flavor.

Protein is my favorite nutrient. It's the best for developing and preserving lean muscle. Keeping muscle is key because muscle is your body's metabolic regulator. Keep in mind that body-mass muscle is living tissue and burns calories like an inferno, so the more muscle on your body, the more calories you burn—both at rest and during exercise. If you want low body fat, you must hold on to as much muscle as possible. Protein helps you do that. There's more: Protein keeps you feeling full and zaps hunger pangs. I'll go into more detail on protein in Chapter 2.

## I DID IT ON DOLVETT'S PROGRAM!

I was pretty amazed because, after the very first day, I lost 2 whole pounds. The second day, I lost another pound, and the third day, another pound. I did my cheat day on the fourth day, and my weight loss briefly stabilized—which was fine because I loved having a break from dieting. I was able to build one of my all-time favorite desserts into my diet—chocolate pie. I did stop drinking soda and learned how to drink more water instead. I really didn't think I'd be able to stick to the diet for long, but after I kept losing so much weight, I became totally committed.

Another habit I changed was skipping breakfast. I always thought I'd lose weight if I went without breakfast and snacks. But that never worked. When Dolvett advised eating all through the day, I thought he was nuts. It seemed like too much food. But my way of dieting had never worked, so I gave his suggestions a try. I also cut back on refined carbs. In the morning I had smoothies. For lunch and dinner, I ate lean proteins and fresh veggies. Well, this all worked, and my weight loss is living proof.

From there, I kept losing, especially after learning and doing Dolvett's workout plan. I challenged myself with the workouts, always striving to do more. Before, I wasn't consistent with exercise. I'd be lucky if I worked out once a week. I felt great after Dolvett's workouts, and I learned that I can push a lot harder than I thought I could. I felt so energized after the workouts that they inspired me to eat very clean during the day. Seeing the results and feeling lighter really motivated me.

At the time of this writing, I've lost 18 pounds and plan to keep this diet and workout program forever. It is perfect for my lifestyle because I never feel deprived. Best of all, though, I think I look amazing!

My tips:

- Make sure your meals have the proper balance of fiber, protein, and carbs. Watch your portions and eat food in moderation. Don't think you have to eat everything on your plate, either. If you're full, stop eating.
- Treat yourself to nonfood items after you have a good week. My treats are shopping for clothes or going to a day spa for a facial or massage. All of these activities make me feel great.

> ■ Get your mind in the right place. I like to visualize what I will look like when I get to my final goal. I see myself slimmer and more fit, walking on the beach in a bikini or walking into a party in a sexy dress. And I start each day visualizing how I will eat healthy and exercise intensely. Visualizations are great fat burners!
>
> —Karina J.

While protein is essential to the growth and preservation of muscle, carbohydrates provide the fuel you need to exercise and go about your daily activities. If your body doesn't have carbohydrates available for energy, it won't hesitate to tap into muscle tissue for energy substrates. The carbs on the clean-eating portion of this diet come from healthy foods like certain types of fruit, starchy vegetables, and high-fiber whole grains.

## SCIENTIFIC SUPPORT

I've been putting clients on this diet for years, so I've seen it work wonders. Allow me to share what I've observed. First—and you won't believe this, but it's true—you can expect to lose up to 1 pound a day the very first week, particularly after your clean-eating days. The second week, you may lose 3 to 4 pounds. From that point forward, your weight loss will be in the range of 2 to 3 pounds a week. When you do my workout routine in conjunction with the diet, your weight loss could be even higher.

Your body is housing a certain amount of fat. At any given moment that fat is being burned or stored. It's never stagnant. Incorporate this diet into your life and get off your tush with my workout, and you'll torch fat more easily and rapidly than you ever thought possible.

My real-life work supports much general research that shows how the body responds to varying caloric intakes and exercising. For example, a study from the Netherlands showed that periodic calorie increases can affect our sympathetic nervous system activity. That's the part of the nervous system mostly involved in stress reactions and metabolism. In plain terms, this study demonstrated that when people changed their calories from low to high and back to low again, their metabolisms ran more efficiently than if they had kept their calories low all the time.

Some other studies show that increasing calories periodically with food helps you put on more lean muscle. How? Well, scientists have found that this style of eating naturally jacks up anabolic hormones (chemicals that help the body repair and build tissue) in your body. On the other side of the coin, research tells us that drastic and continuous calorie cutting (like most diets prescribe) drives down those same hormones. The result? You guessed it: muscle loss and fat gain (which is why a lot of diets erode your muscle tissue). Okay, maybe these studies won't cause you to fall over in amazement. But they do underline the fact that swings in calorie intake can help you get a hot bod.

Your body will respond positively to this diet. It's simple and will fit your lifestyle. It's based on balance and common sense regarding food and getting lean. The 3-1-2-1 Diet is really a long-term eating strategy, not a diet, though I call it one. It allows you to manipulate calories on a weekly basis in order to turn your body into a muscle-building, fat-burning machine—for life.

## AFFIRM TO GET FIRM: YOUR SELF-TALK

I believe that you become what you say you are. How many times have you asked someone, "How are you today?" and you're met with responses such as "Don't ask" or "Terrible." I believe in responding with words like: *great, fantastic, splendid, awesome, brilliant, never felt better,* and so forth. Any other response is unacceptable!

More often than not, the way we talk to ourselves really affects us, holding us back or hurling us forward. How many times have you said to yourself, "I wish I could lose weight," then without even thinking about it, you throw in the towel, believing that the goal is an impossible dream? But this self-talk hurts you in more ways than you realize. It starts to spread like a weed, taking over all parts of your life. Down on yourself, you always expect to fall short of your precious goals.

If you want to transform yourself into an upbeat, positive, energetic, and passionate human being, you can—by becoming what you say you are. Say that you're happy. Say that you're beautiful. Say that you can do whatever you need to do, whether it's losing weight or exercising more. Tell yourself you are what you want to become and you will become it. Then practice it.

# HOW BIG DO YOU WANT TO LOSE?

Goals are important and make everything we want possible. They add energy, direct our lives, and are one of the truly successful techniques in weight control. If you don't know where you're going, how will you get there?

There's a cool goal-setting method you may have heard about: SMART goals. This acronym stands for *specific*, *measurable*, *achievable*, *rewarding*, and *timed*. So first, your goal must be specific; in other words, the more detailed, the better. Saying you'll eat more vegetables is too vague; but saying you'll eat 5 servings of vegetables a day is specific. Consider another example: "I want to get in shape" versus "In 1 month, I want to be able to walk a mile without resting." One is vague, the other specific.

Second, your goal should be measurable—in other words, something you can quantify—such as performing the exercise routine in this book 3 times a week or identifying an ideal weight you'd like to reach and maintain.

Third, make sure your goals are achievable—within your capabilities, genetics, and age. Sure, I'd like to be an NBA pro, but I'm 5 feet, 6 inches so...that's highly unlikely. Likewise, you can't have the bod of a slim eighteen-year-old (unless of course you are eighteen), because our bodies change and tend to lose muscle as they age, and fat tends to shift. (You can begin to reverse this process now by faithfully following the workout in this book.) Remember the realities of genetics when you set weight-loss goals too. If your family is big framed, no program will make you a perfect size 2. Healthier, yes. Trimmer, yes. Tiny, probably not.

Fourth, a goal must be rewarding. What I mean is that there should be a sense of satisfaction and fulfillment tagged to it. What type of goal will truly inspire you? Finishing a 5K race? Fitting into a smaller size?

Finally, goals must be timed. For example, if your goal is to perform my workout the full 48 minutes each time, at least 4 times a week, wear a watch while you walk to track the time, and mark on your calendar the 4 days on which you'll do the workout.

I'll add another criterion here: Make your goals fun and challenging, and choose goals that make you feel good about yourself: Try a new mind/body class this week, experiment with a new recipe, order a salad instead of a fattening appetizer when you eat out, or switch from your midmorning doughnut to a piece of fresh fruit. Put your goal list where you can see it, and before you go to bed at night, think about your goals and how you'll achieve them. We achieve what we believe.

Be sure to test each goal you've written against the SMART criteria, and you'll find yourself piling up successes left and right. Also, if there are specific steps you need to take to make your goals happen, record those too. I call these steps "mini-goals"—daily goals like eating the right foods, exercising, doing daily affirmations, and all that. Mini-goals are steps toward your major goals—those big goals such as reaching your ideal weight or pulling down those bad cholesterol numbers. Look at it this way: A building is built brick by brick. A race is won stride by stride. A picture is painted stroke by stroke. In any program to set new positive habits, it's helpful to make daily manageable resolutions rather than overfocus on far-end goals.

Here are some examples of daily mini-goals:

I will stick to my eating plan today.
I will drink enough water.
I will try one new vegetable today.
I will sprinkle less salt.
I will pay attention to my portion sizes.
I will avoid sugary and fatty foods today.
I will read something inspirational to fuel my mind.
I will do Dolvett's workout.
I will play an active game with my kids.
I will eat a healthy breakfast.
I will practice affirming thoughts.

Do these "I wills" every day, and you *will* get to your ultimate goal!

And listen, everyone: By the time you hit your goal weight, this way of exercising and eating will have become second nature, raising your possibility of successful weight maintenance.

As part of this process, imagine how your life will change after you achieve your goals. Review your goals from time to time, and congratulate yourself for moving forward.

# YOUR IDEAL GOAL WEIGHT

I believe it's vitally important to have a goal weight, or at least a goal range you want to achieve. A lot of people are using a measurement called body mass index, or BMI, to determine goal weights. BMI factors in your height and weight but doesn't take into account the fact that you might be carrying body-shaping muscle. Under BMI calculations, you could be considered fat when you have a curvy, defined, and in-shape physique. So I prefer that you use an old standard to find your goal weight, the Metropolitan Life Insurance weight tables. I've included the tables for women and men below. Look at the tables and pick a realistic weight range for your height. Write it down, then stash it away. Then set your mini-goals to get there.

| Weight Chart for Women | | | |
|---|---|---|---|
| Height | Small Frame | Medium Frame | Large Frame |
| 4'10" | 102–111 | 109–121 | 118–131 |
| 4'11" | 103–113 | 111–123 | 120–134 |
| 5'0" | 104–115 | 113–126 | 122–137 |
| 5'1" | 106–118 | 115–129 | 125–140 |
| 5'2" | 108–121 | 118–132 | 128–143 |
| 5'3" | 111–124 | 121–135 | 131–147 |
| 5'4" | 114–127 | 124–138 | 134–151 |
| 5'5" | 117–130 | 127–141 | 137–155 |
| 5'6" | 120–133 | 130–144 | 140–159 |
| 5'7" | 123–136 | 133–147 | 143–163 |
| 5'8" | 126–139 | 136–150 | 146–167 |
| 5'9" | 129–142 | 139–153 | 149–170 |
| 5'10" | 132–145 | 142–156 | 152–173 |
| 5'11" | 135–148 | 145–159 | 155–176 |
| 6'0" | 138–151 | 148–162 | 158–179 |

| Weight Chart for Men | | | |
|---|---|---|---|
| Height | Small Frame | Medium Frame | Large Frame |
| 5'2" | 128–134 | 131–141 | 138–150 |
| 5'3" | 130–136 | 133–143 | 140–153 |
| 5'4" | 132–138 | 135–145 | 142–156 |
| 5'5" | 134–140 | 137–148 | 144–160 |
| 5'6" | 136–142 | 139–151 | 146–164 |
| 5'7" | 138–145 | 142–154 | 149–168 |
| 5'8" | 140–148 | 145–157 | 152–172 |
| 5'9" | 142–151 | 148–160 | 155–176 |
| 5'10" | 144–154 | 151–163 | 158–180 |
| 5'11" | 146–157 | 154–166 | 161–184 |
| 6'0" | 149–160 | 157–170 | 164–188 |
| 6'1" | 152–164 | 160–174 | 168–192 |
| 6'2" | 155–168 | 164–178 | 172–197 |
| 6'3" | 158–172 | 167–182 | 176–202 |
| 6'4" | 162–176 | 171–187 | 181–207 |

*Ideal weights according to the Metropolitan Life Insurance Company tables.*

## KNOW YOUR FRAME SIZE

At this point, you're probably wondering what your "frame size" is. A lot of people say they have a small frame and don't want to admit that they are, in fact, big boned. So to be really, really accurate, let's figure out your true frame size. First, using a cloth tape measure, measure your wrist just below your wrist bone, which is the smallest point. Next, use the following charts to determine your frame size:

| Women | | |
|---|---|---|
| *Height* | *Wrist Circumference* | *Frame Size* |
| Shorter than 5'2" | Less than 5½" | Small |
| | 5½" to 5¾" | Medium |
| | Over 5¾" | Large |
| 5'2" to 5'5" | Less than 6" | Small |
| | 6" to 6¼" | Medium |
| | Over 6¼" | Large |
| Taller than 5'5" | Less than 6¼" | Small |
| | 6¼" to 6½" | Medium |
| | Over 6½" | Large |

| Men | | |
|---|---|---|
| *Height* | *Wrist Circumference* | *Frame Size* |
| Taller than 5'5" | 5½" to 6½" | Small |
| | 6½" to 7½" | Medium |
| | Over 7½" | Large |

# MORE BENEFITS OF THE 3-1-2-1 DIET

In a matter of weeks, you'll be looking great and feeling great. But the benefits don't stop there. Here's a rundown:

## *Borrrrrrring—NOT!*

You know as well as I do that following a particular diet can be boring, to put it mildly. The 3-1-2-1 Diet is definitely not boring. You have the ability to switch your diet gears and change your eating habits for a little while, and that can give you a tremendous psychological boost.

## Prevent Plateaus

You've probably been on diets before when you hit a plateau and stopped losing weight. Those snags are very frustrating. Many of the *Biggest Loser* contestants experience a weight-loss plateau at some point in the competition. They'll be dropping pounds like crazy for weeks at a time and then suddenly their weigh-in numbers will drop or flatten out. When this happens, I remind my team that the body can plateau but the mind never does. Push yourself! After all, this is a lifestyle. Your body may not do what you want today, but it will react tomorrow! Just keep going.

On this diet, plateaus are less likely, however. Do I hear a collective cheer? When you systemically decrease, then increase, calories, you're confusing your body, and it responds by keeping your metabolic rate high and your body in a losing mode. Translation: fewer plateaus, and nice steady weight loss.

---

### Dolvett's Dos and Don'ts

*Do* count your calories, especially on cheat days.

*Don't* beat yourself up over an imperfect day. Start over at your very next meal.

*Do* drink plenty of water, preferably distilled water (it flushes the body more effectively than other waters). And how much is that? I have a very simple rule: Take half your weight in pounds, convert that number to ounces, and drink that many ounces of water each day. The math is easy. Suppose you weigh 180 pounds. Half of 180 is 90; that means you should drink 90 ounces of water daily, or about eleven 8-ounce glasses of pure $H_2O$.

*Do* make sure you follow my program to the letter. Don't just select the parts you're willing to do…do it all.

*Do* stop eating when you're full, or just before you're full. It takes your body about 20 minutes to get the "full" message from your brain, so slow down and enjoy your food.

*Do* include my exercise routine.

---

## A Permanent Fix

The ugly truth about traditional diets is that most of them fail. Think back with me for a moment about the last time you went on a restrictive diet of deprivation. Do you remember how, when you went off that diet, the fat pounds practically avalanched back?

Here's why: The minute you reintroduce even a bite of "non-diet" food back into your eating, the body responds by packing those calories away as fat. Why? Because that restrictive diet slowed your metabolism to a crawl and tipped your body into a fat-storing mode rather than a fat-burning mode. So for maintaining weight loss, traditional diets will never, ever work. But on my plan, your metabolism is working at fever pitch, burning fat and calories like mad.

# TWO QUESTIONS BEFORE YOU BEGIN

Many people come to me, and I can tell right away that they have a negative attitude. I know they're probably going to fail, because they're taking no responsibility for their weight problem. Just a few weekends ago, I was speaking to a group of ladies. In the question-and-answer period, a woman stood up and said, "I've tried everything, and I just can't lose weight." As nicely as I could, I said, "Sweetheart, you're just not trying hard enough."

Losing weight and getting in shape start with the right attitude. Before you start on the road to weight loss, please answer the following questions:

*How bad do you want it?*

I hope you answered: Really, really bad, and I'm willing to put forth the effort to get it!

Okay, then:

*Will you adopt the 3-1-2-1 Diet as your "final diet"?*

I hope you answered: Yes!

The 3-1-2-1 Diet isn't a diet to get on, then fall off a few months later. It takes a new approach to getting lean, one scientifically based on using food and exercise to tap into your body's hidden potential to burn fat. While unconventional, this plan gives you greater amounts of muscle and less fat than traditional dieting methods.

The best gift of a healthier lifestyle is adding more years to your life while looking and feeling great. But the only way you'll get all the healthy benefits is by living this plan for good. Without question, this is the easiest and best way to live a lean lifestyle and stay trim and fit in the process. You won't be able to read any page of this book without saying "I can do this! I can do this!"

I know you can...so let's do it.

# 2 Eating Clean

You can't be lean unless you eat clean. That means sticking to foods that are unprocessed and close to their natural state most days of the week. Do that, and you'll take off pounds easily and keep them off. And by cutting out the junk and choosing foods that give your body nourishment, you'll feel fuller, even though you're eating fewer calories. You'll also feel more energetic and start easily losing inches, along with the fat.

I think it's fair to say that you've eaten yourself into your weight problem, so now I'm going to show you how to eat yourself out of it. I've written this chapter to give you a much-needed road map to help you find your way back to better nutrition, a healthier lifestyle, and a physique you'll want to show off. Here's how you can clean up your diet and get in amazing shape.

## EAT SMART TO LOSE

The foods on this part of the plan are geared toward helping you strip off body fat and develop lean, toned muscle. So from now on, you're going to ask yourself one question before you eat any food: "Will it help me burn fat?" If your answer is no... well, don't eat it.

Quick review: You'll follow a delicious, "clean" eating plan for 3 days, allow yourself to cheat for 1 day, eat clean again for 2 days, and reward yourself with a cheat meal the next day. There are few foods that are off-limits, and you'll never feel deprived on this eating plan. The 3-1-2-1 Diet provides a nourishing mix of proteins, carbohydrates, fats, vitamins, minerals, and water to keep your metabolism running and to help enhance your health.

I'm also very much into teaching people how to eat healthy on a budget. Many people think that eating healthy is too expensive a habit to work into their regular routines, but if you buy your veggies, proteins, nuts, and so forth in bulk from a big-box store like Costco or Sam's Club, you'll find that it's remarkably inexpensive to eat healthy and save money. I've got more money-saving tips to share throughout this chapter as I review with you what foods to eat on your clean days. So right now, let's talk about those foods.

## Smart Proteins

Hands down, protein is the best type of "diet" food. For anyone who's overweight, eating more protein will help you burn fat more efficiently and speed up your weight loss. I see this with my *Biggest Loser* team all the time when they start eating more protein. Typically, folks with weight problems tend to burn fat sluggishly, but in a study published in the journal *Nutrition & Dietetics*, researchers discovered that higher-protein diets stepped up fat burning in overweight volunteers. The reason? Protein has a higher thermic effect of food than other foods. The thermic effect of food is a measurement of the heat it takes to burn calories. Protein takes a lot of heat to burn, and that means more calories are burned to process it, and ultimately more body fat is burned off.

How many calories can you expect to burn by eating protein at meals? Researchers at Arizona State University looked into this, and I love what they discovered. They compared people who ate either a high-protein or a high-carbohydrate diet, then measured their rate of calorie burn several hours after each meal. The calorie burn was nearly 100 percent higher on the high-protein diet in contrast to the high-carbohydrate diet. That difference amounted to an extra 30 calories burned per meal! What does that mean to you? Well, let's say you eat three main meals a day. That means you could burn an extra 90 calories a day, automatically. I sure like the idea that eating food helps me burn calories, don't you?

Protein acts like a natural appetite suppressant too. It fills you up longer than carbs do. I can explain the reason to you by reviewing the carb-to-energy process. After you eat carbs, they're broken down into your bloodstream as glucose (blood sugar). To get into cells for energy, glucose requires an escort: the hormone insulin. Insulin takes glucose from your bloodstream into your cells. At that point, your blood sugar falls, and you start feeling hungry. Protein, by contrast, doesn't break down into glucose after you eat. It breaks down into amino acids. Amino acids don't affect insulin or its action. In fact, they have a stabilizing effect on glucose and insulin—which means your hunger levels aren't as influenced as they are when you eat carbs.

You'll store less fat on a higher-protein diet too. Protein and carbs may have the same amount of calories (4 per gram), but they act differently in the body. Carbs are more likely to be packed away as fat because some carbs are loaded with simple sugars. Those sugars spike glucose levels, triggering a flood of insulin to bring glucose down. That reaction causes calories to be stored as fat. I will caution you, however: Eat too many of either carbs or protein, and any excess calories are packed away as body fat.

One of my requirements on this plan is that you do my exercise program. It will help you build lean muscle and burn unsightly fat. Eating plenty of protein, on top of exercising, can help you preserve the muscle you already have and develop more.

On my diet, you'll be getting a good deal of your daily protein from fish, and that's a good thing for weight loss. Fish provides a surprising weight-loss perk. It shrinks fat cells and enhances fat loss by raising the amount of leptin in your body. You've probably heard of leptin. It's a hormone made in fat cells that regulates appetite and metabolism. With high levels of leptin, you don't feel hungry, and your metabolism runs normally.

There's more to love about fish. It's loaded with omega-3 fatty acids. These fat particles help jack up serotonin, a feel-good brain chemical in your body. What does that mean to you? It means a better mood—and bad moods and depression cause a lot of people to overeat and binge on fattening comfort foods. If you're in a good mood, feeling good about yourself, you're more likely to stick to the plan.

Have I convinced you that protein is your secret weight-loss weapon? I hope so. Now here's a list of Smart Proteins you'll eat on this part of my plan.

## Smart Proteins

### Fish

| | |
|---|---|
| Canned light tuna (in water) | Salmon |
| Catfish | Sole |
| Flounder | Tilapia |

Be choosy about fish. Wild-caught is better than farm-raised fish, which may have been dosed with antibiotics. And larger fish such as swordfish, shark, king mackerel, and albacore tuna may harbor toxic metals like mercury.

### Shellfish

| | |
|---|---|
| Clams | Oysters |
| Crab | Scallops |
| Mussels | Shrimp |

### Poultry

| | |
|---|---|
| Chicken breasts | Turkey bacon, reduced-fat |
| Eggs (2 eggs = 1 serving) | Turkey breasts |
| Egg whites (4 egg whites = 1 serving) | Turkey ham, fat-free |
| Turkey, lean ground | |

*The serving size for fish and poultry proteins, unless otherwise specified, is 4 ounces, about the size of a deck of cards.*

### Vegetable Proteins

Beans and legumes (black beans, black-eyed peas, butter beans, garbanzo beans, great northern beans, kidney beans, lentils, lima beans, navy beans, peas, pinto beans, split peas, white beans)

*The serving size for vegetable proteins is ½ cup for women; 1 cup for men.*

These are great protein choices if you're a vegetarian or vegan and choose to follow a plant-based diet.

### Other Proteins

Almond milk (1 cup = 1 serving)
Coconut milk (1 cup = 1 serving)
Cottage cheese, low-fat (1 serving = ½ cup)

Yogurt (1 serving = 1 cup)

Protein powders (whey, brown rice, hemp) (1 scoop = 1 serving)

Protein powders are terrific choices for making smoothies.

---

### Smart Shopping Tips for Smart Proteins

- Buy large bags of frozen chicken and fish. They're often cheaper than the same proteins in fresh form, but be sure to compare prices first.
- Save some bucks when purchasing poultry, which is high in protein, by buying a whole turkey or chicken. Whole chickens, turkeys, and some fish are cheaper uncut.
- Love those legumes. From beans to lentils, legumes are not only nutritious; they're supereconomical, high in protein, and loaded with vitamins, minerals, and fiber.
- Check the meat counter for manager's specials and the meat markdown bin.
- Think "soup" before you throw leftovers away. Freeze bones, and when you have enough, prepare stock by boiling them in water for about an hour. Toss in some white-meat chicken or beans for protein, plus veggies, herbs, and brown rice, and you've got a hearty, nutritious meal.

---

## Smart Fibers (Vegetables and Greens)

Anybody interested in tight abs? Ah, I thought so. One way you can get them is to amp up the fiber in your diet. Fiber shrinks belly fat. A study I read by researchers at Wake Forest Baptist Medical Center shows that one way to burn belly fat is easy: Eat more soluble fiber from vegetables, along with fruit and beans. The research discovered that for every 10-gram increase in veggie fiber eaten per day, belly fat shrunk by 3.7 percent over 5 years. (Ten grams is the amount of fiber you'd get from eating 1 medium apple and 1 cup of steamed broccoli.)

Eating fiber also helps prevent constipation. Fiber helps push food through the small intestines, thereby getting rid of waste. (It's hard to have flat abs if your pipes are backed up.)

I'm a huge fan of fiber, even though it isn't much of a nutrient. It's the part of plant foods that can't be digested, so it passes through our bodies without being metabolized. But it does provide bulk. That's another reason why it's a great addition to your diet when you're trying to lose weight. High-fiber foods also stay in your stomach longer than other foods, keeping the feeling of fullness around and delaying the return of hunger.

Fiber—you just gotta love it. The foods in the list below, which include vegetables and certain fruits, are high-fiber goodies you'll be eating on this diet. By the way, the more colorful the fruit or vegetable, the more nutritious. So put a lot of color on your plate. In general, this color rule is a good one to follow, but even white veggies like cauliflower are healthy options too.

### Smart Fibers (Vegetables and Greens)

Alfalfa sprouts
Artichokes
Artichoke hearts
*Asparagus
*Bell peppers, green, red, orange,
    and yellow
*Broccoli
Broccoli sprouts
*Brussels sprouts
*Cabbage
Cauliflower
*Celery
*Cucumbers
Eggplant
Garlic
*Green, leafy vegetables (beet greens,
    turnip greens, collard greens)

*Green beans
*Kale
*Lettuce, all varieties
Mushrooms
*Okra
Onions
*Parsley
Radishes
*Scallions
*Spinach
Summer squash
Swiss chard
Tomatoes
*Watercress
Yellow wax beans
Zucchini

*The serving size for vegetables is ½ to 1 cup.*

## Honorable Mention: Green Fibers

The foods I've marked with an asterisk are "greens." Enjoy them liberally—eat as much of them as you want! That's because greens are the number one food you can eat a lot to help improve your health and boost weight loss. They're full of fiber, along with vitamins, minerals, and phytochemicals (health-giving substances that help protect you from heart disease, diabetes, and even cancer). Plus, greens are natural diuretics. They help flush excess water out of your body. No more ugly bloating or puffiness standing in the way of looking your best as you drop pounds.

My favorite greens are the leafy type. I'm talking lettuce, spinach, kale, mustard greens, beet greens, collard greens, and others like those. They're super sources of vitamins A and C and other nutrients (including calcium, iron, and fiber) and are low in calories and sodium. While great to eat raw, they're also delicious cooked. A mess of greens—sautéed in a little olive oil with garlic, red peppers, and maybe a splash of soy sauce or Italian dressing—is terrific. I also like to stir fresh spinach into omelets and soups, not only for flavor but also for the nutritional boost it provides.

One of the best ways to get your greens is to toss them into a smoothie. A handful of spinach, for example, tastes great blended into a frozen mixture of bananas and berries. Add green leafy vegetables to just about any smoothie, especially those made with blueberries, blackberries, or raspberries. Berries are super-high in antioxidants and fiber and low in calories and sugar, making them a fantastic food for weight loss.

### *Fibrous Fruits*

Apples
Berries, all types
Cherries
Grapefruit
Peaches
Pears
Plums

*The serving size for fibrous fruits is 1 piece of fruit or 1 cup of chopped fruit.*

| Smart Shopping Tips for Smart Fibers |
|---|

- Buy produce in season to save money and enjoy it at its most delicious and nutritious. Fruits and vegetables usually cost less when they're in season. A good source of economical, in-season produce is your local farmers' market. Go-to foods such as apples, bananas, broccoli, lettuce, and spinach are typically priced right year-round.
- Use your freezer. Some fruits and vegetables freeze so they last longer. Bananas freeze well, for example, and are fantastic in smoothies. A lot of people freeze grapes and eat them frozen too, like candy.
- Grow your own vegetable garden. Even if all you have room for is a pot on your apartment balcony, fill it with a tomato plant, pepper plants, or herbs and enjoy fresh vegetables dirt cheap, literally.
- Fresh is great, but it's okay to use canned foods. Here's why: Some canned foods have even higher nutrient levels than fresh. Two good examples are canned tomatoes and canned carrots. Canned tomatoes are higher in a cancer-fighting substance called lycopene than fresh tomatoes are; and canned carrots are higher in beta-carotene than raw carrots are.
- Compare the costs of fresh, canned, and frozen to see which one costs less. Buy canned vegetables that are labeled sodium-free or reduced sodium, and look for sale items.
- Consider store or discount brands. They're usually cheaper while still providing comparable quality.

## Smart Carbs

On to carbs... But before you lump all carbs into one dieting evildoer category, hear me out. Carbohydrates are simply the sugars and starches found in our food. They're important because your body needs these sugars to burn as fuel. The problem with carbs, though, is that if you eat too many of them, they get stored in your fat cells. And once they hole up there, they're almost impossible to boot out.

I broadly divide carbs into Smart Carbs and Cheat Carbs. What makes a carb a Cheat Carb? When it hangs in the wrong places—in this case, at processing machines that strip away most of its beneficial fibers and nutrients. When carbs are processed, they more readily release their sugars. These sugars cause a rapid spike in insulin, which is needed to quickly metabolize the sugars, but you're left feeling empty (and hungry) as soon as that fuel is burned. And keep in mind, insulin is a fat-storing hormone, so you don't want to spike it.

Cheat Carbs are foods like white bread, white rice, white pasta, and anything made with white sugar or flour. White bread is a rather bad Cheat Carb, by the way. Researchers at Tufts University measured the waistlines and analyzed the diets of 459 people. Lo and behold, they discovered that, even in men of similar ages and exercise levels, those who were big white-bread eaters were typically heavier than those who didn't eat much white bread. The researchers suspect that somehow, the calories from white bread just seem to camp out at the belly more than calories from other foods.

Most processed foods that are white (especially if they have to be "enriched") got that way because they were literally bleached of the nutritional benefits they once had. White potatoes, though natural, are Cheat Carbs, because they get digested too quickly in the body—a reaction that can cause an insulin spike. All that said, I call them Cheat Carbs because you get to eat them on your cheat days, but in moderation, of course.

Smart Carbs, on the other hand, are those that come to us in their pure, natural form—unprocessed. The body has to work harder to break down Smart Carbs. A slow breakdown slows insulin production, stabilizes blood sugar, and makes you feel fuller longer. The net effect: Smart Carbs help you get rid of fat rather than store it.

I put Smart Carbs into three categories. First, fruit carbs include those foods that are a little higher in natural starches and sugars. Bananas are a good example. Second, vegetable carbs include those that are starchier, but still digest slowly, such as beets and sweet potatoes. And finally, gluten-free or low-gluten starches include gluten-free multigrain bread and certain whole grains such as brown and wild rice. They're not only free of gluten but also free of sodium, cholesterol, and trans fat. Plus they're nonallergenic, easy to digest, and nutrient packed, with more than fifteen vitamins and minerals. Quinoa is another gluten-free example. Both quinoa and brown or wild rice make better side dishes for weight loss than turn-to-fat mashed potatoes or white rice.

I do prefer that you eat gluten-free foods, even if you're not sensitive to gluten (the offending protein in many starches). If you go mostly gluten-free, you'll have less digestive bloating, more energy, and better mental focus. Even though gluten-free diets are not weight-loss diets per se, I've seen them stimulate weight loss in a lot of people, so I'm a believer.

### Fruit Carbs

| | | |
|---|---|---|
| Apricots | Mangoes | Peaches |
| Bananas | Melons | Pineapples |
| Grapes | Oranges | Watermelon |
| Kiwis | Papayas | |

*The serving size for fruit is 1 piece, 1 cup of grapes, or 1 cup of chopped fruit.*

### Vegetable Carbs

| | |
|---|---|
| Beets | Sweet potatoes |
| Carrots | Winter squashes (acorn, spaghetti, butternut) |
| Parsnips | |
| Pumpkins | Yams |

*The serving size for vegetables carbs is 1 beet, 1 carrot (or ½ cup cooked carrots), 1 to 2 parsnips, ½ cup pumpkin, 1 medium yam or sweet potato, 1 cup mashed squash, and ½ acorn squash.*

### Starchy Carbs

| | |
|---|---|
| Bread, multigrain, gluten-free | Whole grains, other gluten-free (millet, buckwheat, amaranth) |
| Brown rice | |
| Oatmeal | Wild rice |
| Quinoa | |

*The serving size for starchy carbs is 1 slice of bread (women) or 2 slices (men); and ½ cup (women) or 1 cup (men) of brown rice, oatmeal, quinoa, whole grains, or wild rice.*

## Smart Shopping Tips for Smart Carbs

- Look for deals on day-old whole-grain breads. Freeze the loaves.
- Buy nonperishable food items, such as rice and oatmeal, in bulk.
- Purchase store brands of grains such as oatmeal and rice. They're much cheaper than the brand-name versions.

## Smart Fats

Here we come to a topic that's highly controversial in nutrition: fats and how much of them to eat. We definitely need some fat. Fat helps balance blood-sugar levels; is essential for serotonin, a brain chemical that battles depression and controls food cravings; and has a hand in conserving muscle. The downside of fat is that it's high in calories. All fats contain 9 calories per gram. This means you've got to eat some fat, but in small amounts, no more than 1 to 2 tablespoons per day.

My three recommended fats are flaxseed oil, olive oil, and avocado. But let me add my two cents here and explain why this trio is monumentally important.

Flaxseed oil provides *Mega*-nutrition with a capital *M*. It is an excellent source of omega-3 fatty acids. Healthwise, it helps prevent muscle inflammation and provides protection against heart disease and cancer. Nutrition experts value flaxseed oil because it makes you feel fuller than any other oil. This oil is digested more slowly than other foods, so it remains in your stomach longer. There, it helps churn out lots of cholecystokinin, a hard-to-pronounce hormone that signals the brain to stop eating. As a result, digestion slows down and you need less food to feel satisfied. Other studies point out that the omega-3 fatty acids in flaxseed oil fire up your metabolism for greater fat burning.

You can enjoy flaxseed oil in a number of ways: Spread it on your toast, use it in salad dressings, mix it into yogurt, or blend it with smoothies. Flaxseed oil has a sweet, nutty flavor, but it's perishable, so you must keep it in your refrigerator. It's not a good fat to cook with, because heat destroys the omega-3 content. I recommend that you add flaxseed oil to your foods after they've been cooked. I love it on my salads.

On to olive oil. This powerful oil contains an omega-9 oil called oleic acid, which makes up about 80 percent of the oil. For the record, almonds contain oleic acid too. Oleic acid is great for cardiovascular health. It lowers levels of harmful LDL cholesterol and increases levels of protective HDL cholesterol. And it blocks the buildup of fat and plaque in your arteries.

You can cook with olive oil, plus add it to salads and vegetables. Here's something cool: When you add olive oil to tomato-based recipes, the oil soups up the protective power of lycopene, an antioxidant in tomatoes that may help protect again heart disease and cancer. The best type of olive oil is the extra-virgin variety. It contains all the fatty acids and antioxidants found in the olives from which it is made.

Avocado is technically a fruit, but it's high in healthy fat and nutrients like vitamin E. People who regularly eat avocados tend to be at their healthy weights and have small waistlines. That's a pretty good endorsement for including avocados in your diet. I like to mash an avocado with a little lemon juice and use it as a sandwich spread in place of fattening mayo.

You can use these fats with your food, or, in the case of olive oil, it can be used as a cooking oil (but be sure to count it in your daily fat serving).

Avocado, mashed

Flaxseed oil

Olive oil

## Smart Condiments

To perk up flavor, I've got a list of condiments and seasonings for you. Again, be smart here. There are a bunch of condiments that will work in your metabolic favor and keep your fat-burning furnace running. Here's a rundown:

*Vinegar and lemon juice.* Studies show that acidic foods work like lighter fluid, increasing carb combustion by 20 to 40 percent. Researchers believe the acids prevent insulin spikes and slow the rate at which food exits your stomach (which helps you feel full longer). Make your own salad dressings with vinegar or lemon juice, mixed with olive oil or flaxseed oil, and you've got a great weight-control topping for your salads.

*Hot spices and hot sauce.* Cayenne pepper and other spicy foods are fat burners. Why? Because they help boost your metabolism. Cayenne pepper contains capsaicin, a compound that makes the body generate heat in a process known as thermogenesis. Thermogenesis, in turn, helps you burn calories and excess body fat. Studies hint that other hot spices, such as black and white pepper, garlic, and mustard, do the same, even without exercise. (Hold it: Don't take that fact as a license to not exercise. You *do* want to exercise on this plan.) I like to spice my foods liberally for the potential fat burn, plus spices take away my desire for salty foods.

*Ginger.* This spice turns up the heat to naturally boost metabolism. It also helps you feel full. Ginger tastes great on steamed veggies like kale.

*Honey.* This natural sweetener has been studied recently for its effect on appetite. Good news: It acts like an appetite suppressant and may zap cravings. I wouldn't go overboard with honey, though. It's high in calories. Enjoy no more than a tablespoon a day, if you choose to include honey in meals or cook with it.

*Other condiments.* Here are some additional condiments you may use in moderation:

Jams, sugar-free

Ketchup, reduced-sugar

Marinara sauce, low-carb

Salad dressing, fat-free or light

Salsa

Salt substitutes (like Mrs. Dash)

Sour cream, fat-free

Soy sauce, lite

Truvía (a noncaloric sweetener made from natural ingredients)

Vegetable cooking spray

## I DID IT ON DOLVETT'S PROGRAM!

I lost weight right away on the diet: 10 pounds in 12 days. What amazed me was the energy I had. My energy levels were through the roof—which was great since I'm a wife and have two kids to keep up with.

Prior to losing weight, I felt uncomfortable going to the gym. I was too embarrassed to put my body on display. I hated the way I looked. If the subject of exercise came up, I walked away from the conversation. But after I started losing pounds so well, my self-esteem improved and I had the courage to work out at the gym. It was a women-only gym, where I felt less self-conscious. I could adapt Dolvett's workout easily there too. I found that I loved strength training. It made me feel athletic, and before long, I was really looking forward to my workouts. On days when I couldn't make it to the gym because of my children's activities, I'd do the workout at home.

I recorded my meal plans every day. This really helped me stay on track and made me less likely to deviate from the plan. By the end of the first month, I had lost

7 more pounds—so that was a total of 17 pounds in just 1 month. The weight loss really motivated me to keep going.

I continued to lose 2 to 3 pounds a week, without plateaus. I stayed on the plan for 6 months and lost 45 pounds. I'm maintaining now. I'm so happy with the way I look and feel. I do not want to regain that weight. My lifestyle has totally changed and I plan to keep it that way.

My tips:

- Eat slowly. You hear this advice all the time, but it really works. Put your fork down between bites. Take sips of water. Chew your food thoroughly. You'll be surprised at how full you'll feel.
- Enjoy your workouts. Find ways to make exercising fun: Listen to music while you work out, exercise with a friend, or find an upbeat dance exercise class that you like.
- Don't be afraid of sweets. Just manage them with an occasional indulgence on your cheat days. I tried to deprive myself of sweets for years; deprivation made me crave sweets even more and I binged on them as a result. You can enjoy a treat once in a while and still lose weight.

*—Ellen M.*

# SOME ABSOLUTES

There are some bad things that I want you to avoid while eating clean. I call them "absolutes." Let's talk about them now.

## Corn

I never eat corn. I refuse to put anything in my body that can be broken down and put in my gas tank as an alternative fuel to drive my car. And get this: Corn is also used as a base to make glue. Imagine what its glue-like properties might be doing to your insides! Scientists are trying to figure out how to turn corn into lubricants, solvents, fabric, and other industrial stuff. And studies have found that corn takes longer to break down in the body than meat does. So tell me, how can corn be good for you? It's an absolute in my book: Don't eat corn.

## Added Sugar and Sodas

Another absolute is sugar, but not all sugar. Sugars are divided into two main groups: those that occur naturally in foods such as fruit and the added sugar dumped into food and drinks by manufacturers. The natural sugars in fruits are better for you because they're accompanied by fiber and other nutrients. These are more slowly digested and stabilizing and therefore a better choice than added sugars.

Added sugars are a sponge to collect fat. If you want to have fat roaming around in your body, eat that kind of sugar. A high-sugar diet can set you up for heart attacks and strokes by hiking the levels of triglycerides (unhealthy fats) in your blood. These bad fats clog the arteries in much the same way cholesterol does. Added sugar also makes us fat. When you eat sugary foods, your body responds by producing lots of insulin, and that can mean weight gain.

Added sugars add calories too. I'll bet you can't guess how much sugar people eat in a day on average. Answer: 22.2 teaspoons, or 355 calories, *per day*! That astronomical sum tallies up to an annual weight gain of nearly 40 pounds of blubber.

If you're among the sugar devotees, you've got to cut back. Get good at deciphering which foods are most likely to be laced with added sugars. Sugar often lurks in packaged and processed foods, especially those made with white flour and fat. Everything from salad dressings, sweets, and cereals to frozen dinners, pasta sauces, and yogurts contains added sugar. Read the ingredients on the labels of the food you buy. If you find these sugars on the label, I highly recommend avoiding them:

| | | |
|---|---|---|
| Agave nectar | Evaporated cane juice | Maltodextrin |
| Brown sugar | Fructose | Maltose |
| Cane crystals | Glucose | Malt syrup |
| Corn sweetener | High-fructose corn syrup | Raw sugar |
| Corn syrup | Invert sugar | Sucrose |
| Crystalline fructose | Lactose | Sugar |
| Dextrose | Levulose | Syrup |

One of the worst added sugars is high-fructose corn syrup, found largely in sugary soft drinks. One 12-ounce can of soda contains around 150 calories and at least

10 teaspoons of sugar, mostly in the form of high-fructose corn syrup. A single soda per day can equate to a 1-year weight gain of 15 pounds.

I know from research that this rather nasty sugar is destined to end up around your belly. Solid evidence for this came in 2009. In a 10-week study, researchers gave thirty-two overweight or obese middle-aged men and women 25 percent of their calories from beverages laced with either fructose or glucose. Both groups gained the same amount of weight (about 3 pounds). But their new fat didn't all land in the same place. The fructose eaters gained most of that fat in their bellies.

I'm veering a bit off the subject here, but you're probably wondering about diet sodas. They're the lesser of two evils, I suppose. But too many people order diet soda with burgers and fries as if it were somehow going to magically make up for the other fattening calories. Or they argue that, by drinking diet sodas, they get more than the

| Sugar Content in Common Foods | |
|---|---|
| *Food* | *Sugar Content per Serving* |
| Bran flakes, 1 serving | 5 teaspoons |
| Corn flakes, 1 serving | 2 teaspoons |
| Dried fruit, 1 handful | 3 teaspoons |
| Granola bar | 5 teaspoons |
| Mashed potatoes from a box, 1 cup | 8 teaspoons |
| Orange juice, 1 cup | 3 teaspoons |
| Soda, 12 ounces | 12 teaspoons |
| Special K cereal, 1 serving | 4 teaspoons |
| Sports drink, 1 serving | 4 teaspoons |
| Sweetened iced tea, 1½ cups | 8 teaspoons |
| White bread, 1 slice | 4 teaspoons |
| White rice, 1 bowl | 9 teaspoons |
| White wine, 1 glass | 1 teaspoon |
| Yogurt, low-fat fruit flavored, 8 ounces | 7 teaspoons |

*Adapted from USDA data and food labels.*

### Agave Nectar: What's the Real Deal?

People in the fitness industry, including me, used to recommend a popular sweetener called agave nectar. Not so much anymore, though. Agave nectar is fast falling out of favor, and here's why: Agave nectar, like its relative tequila, is made from the agave plant. To make the nectar, manufacturers put the plant through a lengthy refining process to break down the carbohydrates into sugars. So the end product is not exactly as "natural" as it claims to be; it's highly processed. In fact, it's chemically refined fructose and very similar to high-fructose corn syrup. It's true that agave nectar causes less of a blood-sugar spike than other sweeteners; however, the fructose in it can lead to mineral depletion, hardening of the arteries, insulin problems, heart disease, and obesity. Agave nectar is not all it's cracked up to be, so I no longer recommend it. If you want a truly natural sweetener, use honey. I can go right to a beehive and dip out the honey, which I can eat without processing it. It is not refined in the least.

recommended eight glasses of H$_2$O a day. But just because your *aqua* comes carbonated and includes a few fine ingredients like caramel color, phosphoric acid, potassium benzoate, phenylalanine, and other barely pronounceable additives, sodas don't count toward your eight-glasses-a-day quota. Plus, the latest word from research experts is that diet soda may still make you fat. They have come up with data showing that the chemicals in diet soda actually stimulate hunger and sugar cravings and ultimately increase the amount of food people wolf down.

I've heard that you can use soda to clean toilets and even remove rust—now, those are reasons for buying soda that I endorse. As a beverage, it's the worst choice. You can reserve it for your cheat days, if you must. Just make sure it fits into your calorie allotment. But really, wouldn't you rather *eat* something extra that is 150 calories than drink those calories? I certainly would.

## Fast Food

Moving on, my next absolute is fast food. I'm often asked, "Dolvett, can I still eat fast food?" My answer is "No, fast food can kill you." The ingredients in fast food can mess with the way your body works, or doesn't work. On season 14 on *The Biggest Loser*, we tackled the issue of childhood obesity. Through this experience, I learned that in recent years the number of kids and teens under nineteen who are diagnosed with type 2 diabetes is going through the roof. Why? Diabetes is an obesity-related illness, and 15 percent of young people are overweight—which is three times the rate it was in 1980. And one huge reason they're overweight is because they eat so much fast food.

Here's something else you need to know. Fast food isn't just bad for you—it's like a drug, addictive. It's made up of a blend of sugar, fat, and salt, all the stuff we humans love to eat. But while we're feeding our faces, we're filling our arteries with fat and our bodies with refined, added sugar. And we eat so much of this junk because we get conditioned to crave the alluring taste and smell of fast food. And then that's all we want! If I work with someone who leans on fast-food joints and is addicted to that food, I will tell them to stay out of those places—just like I'd tell a recent ex-smoker to stay away from smoking sections.

And just think: If you quit hitting fast-food joints, you'll actually be able to see your car's floors, seats, and dashboard instead of a big pile of old burger wrappers and French fry containers.

Now, here's an exception to this absolute: Most fast-food places, in their defense, do offer healthy choices, such as grilled chicken sandwiches, salads, oatmeal, and apple slices. If you've got to eat on the run, or you're traveling, or you're with your kiddos, hitting the drive-through is fine; just promise yourself that you'll order the healthier menu items.

Fast food—you've just got to give it up (except the healthy choices!). Get addicted to a healthy lifestyle instead.

## Salt and Sodium

Then there is salt. We need some salt or sodium, which is a mineral, because it helps muscles and nerves work properly. It also helps regulate and maintain normal water and blood-volume levels. But there is a big downside to excessive sodium: high blood pressure, or hypertension, which can lead to heart disease and stroke.

Another downside is water retention, which interferes with fat burning. Here's why: Your kidneys need a good supply of water to do their main job efficiently—processing waste products. If they don't get this water (because it's being retained), your liver pinch-hits to help out. Because the liver is responsible for taking your stored fat and burning it for energy, you slow this process down by relying on your liver to process waste products. You can therefore maximize fat loss by making sure your body doesn't retain water and letting your liver do its job of turning that unwanted fat into energy.

There's a lot of sodium hidden in foods too. Check the ingredient list on food labels for the word *sodium*. Sodium goes by other names too, so watch out for products containing the following:

■ Disodium phosphate
■ Monosodium glutamate, or MSG (often added to Asian dishes)
■ Sodium benzoate
■ Sodium caseinate
■ Sodium citrate
■ Sodium hydroxide
■ Sodium sulfite

We Americans, who for the most part like well-salted foods, take in two to four times more sodium than needed. So I advocate just cutting it out altogether. If you think you cannot live without extra salt on your food, here is some encouraging news: Our taste for salt is both acquired and reversible. As you begin to use less salt on your foods, your taste for it will begin to vanish. You can naturally begin to reduce your sodium intake by consuming fresh foods over processed foods (which are loaded with salt) and by knowing what *low sodium* means on food labels. Here's some information to help you decode those labels.

## My Sodium Dictionary

*Unsalted:* No sodium has been added to the food; however, it may contain sodium naturally.

*Sodium-free:* A serving has fewer than 5 milligrams of sodium.

*Very low sodium:* A serving contains 35 milligrams or less of sodium.

*Low sodium:* A serving has 140 milligrams or less of sodium.

*Reduced sodium:* The product contains 25 percent less sodium than it normally contains. If you're watching your sodium intake, this might still be too much for you.

## Sodium Shockers

*In January 2011, the USDA announced dietary guidelines recommending that healthy adults limit their sodium intake to 2,300 milligrams of sodium a day, while people with high blood pressure should consume no more than 1,500 milligrams a day. Consistently consuming more than the recommendation may lead to high blood pressure, and that increases your risk for heart disease, stroke, kidney disease, and congestive heart failure. While eating healthy, I encourage you to pay attention to the sodium content in the foods you choose because some seemingly healthy foods are higher in sodium than you may think.*

| Food | Sodium Content |
|------|----------------|
| American cheese, singles, 1 slice | 277 mg |
| Chicken bouillon, 1 cube | 740 mg |
| Cottage cheese, ½ cup | 360 mg |
| Diet supplement drinks, 1 can | 460 mg |
| Diet TV dinners, 1 meal | 690 mg |
| Dill pickle, 1 | 880 mg |
| Garden burger, 1 | 576 mg |
| Ketchup, 1 tablespoon | 190 mg |
| Light Italian dressing, 2 tablespoons | 440 mg |
| Nut butter, 2 tablespoons | 125 mg |
| Pasta sauce, ½ cup | 510 mg |
| Pumpernickel bread, 1 slice | 190 mg |
| Raisin Bran, 1 serving | 350 mg |
| Salt, 1 teaspoon | 2,000 mg |
| Sauerkraut, 1 cup | 940 mg |
| Soup, canned, 1 cup | 600 mg |
| Whole wheat bread, 1 slice | 260 to 400 mg |

*Adapted from USDA data and food labels.*

In addition, reduce your use of certain sodium-rich condiments, such as soy sauce and ketchup. Finally, learn to cook with, and enjoy, herbs and spices. Both supply added flavor, and like I said, before long, you won't miss the salt. The recipes you'll try in this book are low in sodium, and you'll be surprised at how delicious they taste. You're going to get enough sodium from vegetables anyway. And you'll be a lot healthier for it.

## Soy Products

And, finally, stay away from soy products, mainly soy milk, tofu, soy cheese, and other processed soy foods! They're not health foods, no matter what you hear! Soy has been proven to raise estrogen levels in both men and women. With elevated estrogen levels, your body clings to fat. If you want that to happen, eat soy products. Also, studies have hinted that soy may be implicated in the development of breast cancer. So why would you even consider soy? Soy is a terrible source of protein, terrible. If you want to include a nondairy milk substitute in your diet, reach for almond milk or coconut milk.

---

### AFFIRM TO GET FIRM: HOW YOU DO ANYTHING IS HOW YOU DO EVERYTHING

---

Imagine what might happen if you drove a car halfheartedly, or took care of a child without paying much attention, or worked at a job and did half your best. Or what about the last diet you went on? Did you really give it your all? What was the outcome? Really think about this.

I never do anything half-assed. If there's a way to get results and achieve, I'll find it and do it. The most worthwhile things in life are the most challenging to achieve. That means they involves passion and a commitment to obtain a goal, plus the ability to sustain the passion and commitment. If you don't feel the boundless motivation to achieve something, you may not get there.

I know if you listen to your heart, you'll find that you care about your fitness and health very much. Tap into that desire. Live it, feel it, breathe it every day. Then you can do something many less-motivated people may never do: Stick to the program and achieve the best health and shape of your life.

---

# OTHER ABSOLUTES:
# WHAT NOT TO EAT ON CLEAN DAYS

Alcoholic beverages

Artificial sweeteners, with the exception of Truvía and sugar-free maple syrup (which I recommend when you want syrup on pancakes and waffles but not the calories)

Butter or margarine, or any fats with the exception of avocado, olive oil, and flaxseed oil

Cow's milk

Fast food

Processed, packaged food

Rice milk (this product is very high in carbohydrates)

Salt (use Mrs. Dash or salt substitutes)

Soda, regular or diet

Soy milk and soy products

Sugar in any form, except the sugar that occurs naturally in fruits and vegetables

Syrups, including agave nectar (unless they're sugar-free)

White starches—such as potatoes, white bread, white rice, or white pasta

# HOW MUCH TO EAT—DOLVETT'S DISH

Now we come to the all-important topic of how much to eat. I covered this topic briefly earlier by explaining the general serving size for each type of food. But to simplify all of this, visualize a round dinner plate that is no larger than 10 inches in diameter (the smaller, the better!), divided into three compartments for a Smart Protein, a Smart Fiber, and a Smart Carb. Your Smart Protein covers half of that dinner plate.

The remaining half of the plate should be divided into one compartment for your Smart Fiber and the other for your Smart Carb. And no fair piling those carbs high on the plate. You want about ½ cup (for women) to 1 cup (for men) of carbs. A cup is about the size of your fist; ½ cup is the size of a cupped palm. Plan your meals like this, and you've created what I call Dolvett's Dish. It helps you control portions—but in a very easy way. To reiterate, each meal is a combination of the following nutrients:

1 Smart Protein
1 Smart Fiber
1 Smart Carb

Here are some examples of Dolvett's Dish:

### Breakfast Example 1

4 scrambled egg whites (Smart Protein)
½ tomato, sliced (Smart Fiber)
1 banana (Smart Carb)

### Breakfast Example 2

Smoothie: 1 cup of almond milk + 1 serving/scoop of brown rice protein powder
    (Smart Protein) blended with ½ cup of frozen unsweetened blueberries + handful
    of spinach (Smart Fiber) and 1 to 2 packets of Truvía (optional)
1 to 2 slices of multigrain, gluten-free toast, spread with sugar-free jam (Smart Carb)

### Lunch Example 1

Here's a trick I learned after joining *The Biggest Loser* a few seasons ago: Use lettuce,
rather than bread, to make sandwiches. Sounds funny, but this really tastes great. Here's
a way to make lettuce wraps with chicken salad (which count as 1 Smart Protein, 1
Smart Fiber, and 1 Smart Fat): Dice 1 baked chicken breast. Mix it with 1 tablespoon
of chopped scallion, 2 tablespoons of chopped celery, and 1 tablespoon of olive oil.
Spoon 1 heaping tablespoon of the chicken mixture into the center of 1 big lettuce leaf.
Wrap the leaf around the filling. (We've even done this technique on the show with
burgers.) Serve with a side of ½ cup of cooked quinoa (Smart Carb).

### Lunch Example 2

Lunch salad: 1 baked chicken breast, cut into pieces (Smart Protein) on a liberal
    bed of greens, including salad veggies (Smart Fiber), plus 1 cup of fresh
    pineapple chunks (Smart Carb)
1 to 2 tablespoons of olive oil to drizzle over the salad (Smart Fat)

*Dinner Example 1*

Grilled salmon (Smart Protein)
1 cup of steamed broccoli (Smart Fiber)
1 medium baked sweet potato (Smart Carb)

*Dinner Example 2*

Baked turkey breast (Smart Protein)
1 cup of steamed green beans (Smart Fiber)
½ to 1 cup of brown rice (Smart Carb)

When you combine foods like this and plan your plate accordingly, you automatically take in the correct amount of calories for steady weight loss and fat burning. You don't have to actually count calories on clean days; Dolvett's Dish does it for you.

## I DID IT ON DOLVETT'S PROGRAM!

I was a junk-food addict, for sure. What appealed to me about the 3-1-2-1 Diet was the ability to cheat. It seemed like I could indulge my desire for junk food, namely, Chick-fil-A, and still lose weight, as long as I was careful about it and planned the cheat days into my week. I'm a former gymnast and mother of two, so physical activity was something I was used to. I liked the workout because I could do it on my time—and save time, too.

The first thing I noticed about the diet was that it curbed my appetite, even for junk food. Eating five times a day helped; I was hardly ever hungry. This was the first diet I had tried on which I was not hungry. In fact, I sometimes had trouble getting all my meals in. On cheat days, I would go to my favorite fast-food outlet (although Dolvett doesn't like fast-food places for dieters!) and make good caloric choices that fit within my calorie allotment. The entire diet, from the clean days to the cheat days, was extremely satisfying.

I did have a lot to lose—about 45 pounds. Thinking about all that weight was overwhelming, so I just took things one day at a time. What helped was that I didn't feel like I was dieting, thanks to the cheat days. I'm 10 pounds away from my goal, and I know I'll make it.

My tips:

- Experiment with foods and condiments. I would drizzle honey over plain yogurt and mix it with strawberries. It was just as satisfying as eating ice cream.
- Drink water prior to eating. I got in the habit of drinking a full glass of water before each main meal. It filled me up, plus helped me get in enough water each day.
- Increase the intensity of your workouts. Doing so will help you lose more weight. Lift heavier weights, work out longer, or add more workout days to your week. These are all ways you can burn more fat.

*—Charlotte B.*

# HOW TO SNACK

Snacks are important; you should eat every 2½ to 3 hours. Frequent eating is another way you can keep your metabolism grinding. If you go for more than 3 hours without a meal, your metabolism slows down dramatically and your blood-sugar level drops, leaving you feeling sluggish and craving sugar and starch. A speedy metabolism is what it's all about, baby. Your metabolism gets so charged up that it incinerates any extras calories. Snack on the following:

1 Smart Fiber or Smart Carb fruit or
A handful of almonds or
2 sticks of low-fat string cheese or
A smoothie (see Chapter 5 for recipes) or
1 Smart Fiber vegetable

*Enjoy no more than two snacks a day if you're a woman; two to four snacks a day if you're a man.*

# WORKSHEET FOR DAYS 1, 2, 3, 5, AND 6

While you're on this diet, use the following worksheet to plan your meals. Using the food lists, simply fill in what you will eat each clean day. (You can follow the menus in Chapter 4, if you wish, or create your own, using this worksheet.)

## Breakfast

My Smart Protein: _____

My Smart Fiber: _____

My Smart Carb: _____

Smart Condiments: _____

## Lunch

My Smart Protein: _____

My Smart Fiber: _____

My Smart Carb: _____

Smart Condiments: _____

## Dinner

My Smart Protein: _____

My Smart Fiber: _____

My Smart Carb: _____

Smart Condiments: _____

## Smart Snacks

_____

_____

## Dolvett's Dos and Don'ts for Clean Days

*Do* eat exactly what is outlined.

*Do* rise and grind. Eat breakfast as soon as you get up to start metabolizing. It's true that breakfast is the most important meal of the day. If you eat breakfast, you begin burning calories throughout the day, and you'll be less hungry as the day goes on.

*Do* remove skin from chicken or turkey prior to cooking, or purchase skinless poultry.

*Do* enjoy fresh vegetables and fruits as much as possible. For convenience, frozen and canned items are fine.

*Do* drink distilled water daily in the following manner: Keep a gallon of distilled water handy at all times. Sip it throughout the day: as soon as you get up, after you brush your teeth, with meals, while you're in your car, and so forth. Drink distilled water for the first 2 weeks of the diet; then you can switch to spring water. The point is to stay hydrated throughout the day; doing so will flush toxins from your body and help you lose weight faster. Drink half your weight in water: For example, if you weigh 180 pounds, that's 90 ounces of water daily.

*Do* also hydrate, if you like, with 1 to 2 cups daily of coconut water—particularly after you exercise. Coconut water has more hydration power than water and is lower in calories (45 calories per cup) than sports drinks, making it a great post-workout beverage.

Remember: Snacks are optional; *don't* overdo them or exceed the allowable portions.

*Don't* eat fruit carbs after lunchtime. (When you cut back on fruit after lunch, your body will tap into its fat reserves for energy, and you'll get leaner.)

*Do* eat slowly and only until you're full; do not overload your stomach.

*Do* avoid the foods listed on page 39 (Other Absolutes: What Not to Eat on Clean Days).

*Do* weigh and measure yourself on the following schedule, and record it, so you can keep track of your progress.

# TRACK YOUR PROGRESS

I'd like you to do a few things prior to beginning the program. First, find out how much you weigh. Weigh yourself first thing in the morning before you put on your clothes and shoes. Continue to weigh yourself every few days to give your body time to respond to the program. Record these numbers in a journal, using the form below.

## My Progress in Pounds

Prior to starting the diet: _____

After 3 days: _____

After 7 days: _____

After 14 days: _____

After 21 days: _____

Second, take body-circumference measurements using a cloth tape measure. This simple tool works well for measuring the areas of the body where fat is stored most: the chest, hips, waist, thighs, and upper arms. Write down the measurements for these areas, without your clothes on each time. Keeping a record will help you see how many inches of fat have shrunk away over time. Use the following forms:

## My Progress in Inches

My chest/bust measurement prior to starting the diet: _____

My waist measurement prior to starting the diet: _____

My hip measurement prior to starting the diet: _____

My right thigh measurement prior to starting the diet: _____

My left thigh measurement prior to starting the diet: _____

My upper right arm measurement prior to starting the diet: _____

My upper left arm measurement prior to starting the diet: _____

### After 1 week

My chest/bust measurement: _____

My waist measurement: _____

My hip measurement: _____

My right thigh measurement: _____

My left thigh measurement: _____

My upper right arm measurement: _____

My upper left arm measurement: _____

### After 2 weeks

My chest/bust measurement: _____

My waist measurement: _____

My hip measurement: _____

My right thigh measurement: _____

My left thigh measurement: _____

My upper right arm measurement: _____

My upper left arm measurement: _____

## After 3 weeks

My chest/bust measurement: _____

My waist measurement: _____

My hip measurement: _____

My right thigh measurement: _____

My left thigh measurement: _____

My upper right arm measurement: _____

My upper left arm measurement: _____

Third, ask your doctor for other information, such as your blood pressure and cholesterol readings, based on your annual physical. Record those numbers and watch them improve as you get trimmer and healthier.

Finally, pay close attention to how you feel. Are you walking around feeling good about yourself and your life? If so, great! Write down any and all positive changes, such as better sleep, more stamina, less fatigue, better health, and a feeling of better mental wellness. Take these new outcomes as positive signs of success.

Now that I've shown you how to eat clean, let's turn the tables and talk about what you've been waiting for: how to cheat on your diet. That's where we're headed next.

# 3 Cheat to Lose

Cheat on a diet?

Not just cheat, people—cheat and still lose weight. That's what you get to do twice a week on the 3-1-2-1 Diet.

Think about it: You're doomed to fail if you try to go through life depriving yourself of foods you most enjoy and like to eat the most frequently.

When was the last time you were told that eating your favorite foods was okay and, indeed, a healthy choice? Probably not in a long time, if ever! Looking forward to eating something you really enjoy, such as a slice of pie, is one of life's small pleasures. When you want a treat, have it and enjoy every bite. Then forget it. Just don't have seconds! Oftentimes, when you fight your urge to eat something you really want, your strategy backfires. Think about it: You're doomed to fail if you try to go through life depriving yourself of foods you most enjoy and like to eat the most frequently.

I love carrot cake, for example. I love strawberry shortcake. I love going out and having a drink with my friends. I love my cheat days, period. Dieting is all about balance—not going to extremes.

When you cheat, though, you have to be smart about your choices. I'm not advocating that you tear through a whole box of Krispy Kreme doughnuts or scarf down a whole box of fried chicken at KFC. I am telling you to stay within your calorie count 7 days a week, and this includes more calories on your cheat days. So I am not telling you to cut off the food faucet; I am just saying make it drip.

Your friends will be surprised at what you get to eat too. I was eating dinner one night in an LA restaurant, and someone who recognized me came over and said, "You're a trainer and you're eating pasta? What gives?"

"Just because I'm a trainer doesn't mean I can't eat pasta. Of course, when I eat pasta, I choose whole-grain," I said. "I also eat clean for three days; then I cheat on my fourth day. You just happened to catch me on my fourth day!"

Here's the real kicker: When people see your amazing weight loss, they'll often ask what diet you're on and want to know "What do you eat?"

You can tell them the truth: almost everything and anything. (Just not all in one sitting like you used to. It's all about moderation.) Virtually nothing is off-limits.

Another thing you'll love about this diet is that you're allowed to eat the same foods as your family, particularly on cheat days. The feeling of diet deprivation is strongest while watching your family gobble up pizza or burgers while you nibble on unfamiliar foods or tiny servings. That kind of agony can't go on! With this plan, your family and friends won't even know you're trying to lose weight, unless you tell them.

And while I'm on the subject of family, do others in your family need to drop some pounds? It's very important that, when someone is pursuing a life-changing goal, the people at home join the journey as well. We love the people we love, and they can influence us in one direction or another, sometimes without us even realizing it's happening! A family that diets and sweats together gets together! Building healthy families across the nation is one of the best solutions for a healthier America.

## THE CHEAT DAYS: DAY 4 AND DAY 7

If you're someone who can no longer live without bread, pasta, and other goodies, don't worry about it. You'll be reintroducing foods like these into your diet by following the 3-1-2-1 Diet pattern. That means, each week, eat clean on days 1, 2, 3, 5, and 6 to boost your metabolism and burn fat. (Refer to Chapter 2 for details.)

Then cheat on day 4 and day 7. On both days, you'll get to eat more liberally by incorporating your favorite foods into your meal plan. There is a way to cheat and still keep losing weight, but you still must follow some guidelines (described in this chapter). Physically and psychologically, you need these cheat days to balance your lifestyle with your clean days. The second week, third week, fourth week, and so forth, simply repeat the pattern of 3 clean days, 1 cheat day, 2 clean days, and 1 cheat day—right down to your healthy weight.

# EAT TO CHEAT

Within reason, you can cheat with just about any food in the universe, but for simplicity's sake, I've categorized them for you.

## Cheat Proteins

These are protein-rich foods that might be slightly higher in fat and calories than the ones you eat on clean days, such as your favorite cuts of beef, lamb, pork, or veal. Dark-meat poultry is another example of a cheat protein. How do juicy fall-off-the-bone ribs sound? It doesn't get better than that. You'll still have to watch your portions and calories with these selections or you'll never be able to see your own ribs again. Don't smother cheat proteins with rich sauces, either. They contain a lot of hidden gunk and just aren't healthy.

### *Examples of Cheat Proteins*

Beef
Canadian bacon—2 slices
Fattier cuts of poultry such as chicken thighs, turkey legs, or
    any type of dark-meat poultry
Hard cheeses—2 ounces
Hot dogs—1 dog
Lamb
Luncheon meats—2 slices
Pork
Skim milk—1 cup
Veal

*Unless otherwise noted, the serving size for Cheat Proteins is 4 ounces.*

## Leanest Cuts of Meat

*Good health is part of a happy life. But far too many people are eating themselves to death, one forkful at a time. They gorge on diets high in fat, salt, and calories, all leading to deadly health problems such as diabetes, heart disease, and stroke. Some meats can be among the worst offenders, so I advise folks to choose the leanest meats as their Cheat Proteins. Meat tends to be high in the worst kind of fat, saturated fat. It's the main dietary cause of artery-clogging high blood cholesterol. So one of the best ways you can get fit and trim, and ease back on the amount of cholesterol in your diet, is to choose lower-fat versions of your favorite cheat proteins. By lowering your fat intake, you've got a better chance of fending off heart disease and high blood pressure.*

*The USDA defines a lean cut as about a 4-ounce serving that contains less than 10 grams of total fat, 4.5 grams of saturated fat, and 95 milligrams of cholesterol. An extra-lean cut is a 3.5-ounce serving that contains less than 5 grams of total fat, 2 grams of saturated fat, and 95 milligrams of cholesterol. Here's a look at leanest cuts of meat you can buy.*

### Beef

| Cut | Calories | Total Fat | Saturated Fat |
| --- | --- | --- | --- |
| Sirloin tip side steak | 206 | 5.4 grams | 2.06 grams |
| Top round steak | 240 | 7.6 grams | 3 grams |
| Eye of round steak | 276 | 7 grams | 2.4 grams |
| Bottom round steak | 300 | 11 grams | 3.8 grams |
| Top sirloin | 316 | 10.6 grams | 4 grams |

### Pork

| Cut | Calories | Total Fat | Saturated Fat |
| --- | --- | --- | --- |
| Canadian-style bacon (2 ounces) | 86 | 3.9 grams | 1.3 grams |
| Tenderloin | 163 | 4.8 grams | 1.6 grams |
| Boneless ham, extra-lean | 164 | 4.7 grams | 2.6 grams |
| Boneless loin roast | 147 | 5.3 grams | 2.9 grams |
| Boneless loin chops | 153 | 6.2 grams | 2.2 grams |

### Lamb

| Cut | Calories | Total Fat | Saturated Fat |
| --- | --- | --- | --- |
| Roasted lamb shank | 153 | 2 grams | 5.7 grams |
| Roasted leg of lamb | 162 | 6.6 grams | 2.4 grams |
| Lamb loin | 172 | 8.2 grams | 3.2 grams |

*continued*

| Veal | | | |
|---|---|---|---|
| Cut | Calories | Total Fat | Saturated Fat |
| Top round | 201 | 5 grams | 1.9 grams |
| Leg cutlet | 201 | 5 grams | 1.9 grams |
| Arm steak | 163 | 6 grams | 2.3 grams |
| Sirloin steak | 167 | 6 grams | 2.4 grams |
| Loin chop | 174 | 7 grams | 2.6 grams |

## Cheat Carbs

Ah, carbs! Yes, on cheat days you can replace a Smart Carb with a Cheat Carb. If you're a carb lover, this feature of the diet will be paradise for you. Remember, Cheat Carbs are more processed, with more sugar added, and most of us need to cut back on sugars and starches. So use good judgment, and don't go overboard by planning your meals with too many Cheat Carbs. One or two on your cheat days should be the limit. Follow the recommended portion sizes, and monitor your calories on cheat days.

### Examples of Cheat Carbs

Alcoholic beverages (1 or 2 drinks)

Bagel—1 medium

Crackers—6

Dark chocolate—1 piece, 2" square

Desserts (such as ⅛ of a pie or a 1-inch slice of cake, 1 piece or slice)

Dinner roll—1

Doughnut—1

English muffin—1

Frozen fruit bar—1 bar

Hamburger or hot dog bun—1 piece

Ice cream or frozen yogurt (1 scoop)

Muffin—1

Packaged cold cereals—1 cup

Pancakes or waffles—2 to 3 pieces

Pasta—½ to 1 cup

Potato—1 medium

Reduced-calorie ice cream bar or ice cream sandwich
(such as Skinny Cow products)

Tortilla (flour)—1 to 2

| America's Favorite Desserts | | |
|---|---|---|
| *Is dessert your favorite part of a meal? If you're planning to spend your Cheat Carb calories on dessert, here's a look at how various desserts weigh in, calorie-wise.* | | |
| *Dessert* | *Serving Size* | *Calories* |
| Apple pie | 1 slice, ⅛ of pie (5.5 ounces) | 411 |
| Brownies | 1 slice, 2" square (0.8 ounce) | 112 |
| Carrot cake | 1 slice, ⅙ of cake (2.6 ounces) | 300 |
| Cheesecake | 1 slice, ⅙ of cake (2.8 ounces) | 257 |
| Chocolate cake | 1 piece, ¹⁄₁₂ of cake (4.9 ounces) | 506 |
| Chocolate chip cookies (4) | 2.25" diameter | 192 |
| Fudge, chocolate | 2 pieces, 1" square | 70 |
| Ice cream, vanilla | 1 cup | 473 |
| Jell-O | ½ cup | 70 |
| Pumpkin pie | 1 slice, ⅙ of cake (4.7 ounces) | 279 |

*Source: www.calorieking.com*

## Combination Cheat Proteins and Cheat Carbs

Not every meal can be neatly divided into pure protein or pure carbs. Sometimes you'll eat meals with two or more of these nutrients combined. When foods are combined all in one item, you've got what I call a cheat meal. This is a convenient way to make sure you're combining your protein, carbs, fiber, and fat at meals.

Examples of cheat meals include:

### Meat Pizza

Cheat Protein = Sausage, ham, or pepperoni
Cheat Carb = Pizza crust
Smart Fiber = Vegetables

### Lasagna

Cheat Protein = Beef
Cheat Carb = Pasta
Smart Fiber = Vegetables

### Taco

Cheat Protein = Ground beef
Cheat Carb = Flour tortilla
Smart Fiber = Vegetables

### Beef Stew

Cheat Protein = Beef
Cheat Carb = Potato
Smart Fiber = Vegetables

### Deli Sandwich

Cheat Protein = Roast Beef
Cheat Carb = Sandwich Roll
Smart Fiber = Vegetables
Cheat Fat = Mayo

## *Cheat Fats*

On cheat days, you can be a little more liberal in your fat choices. But again, please watch portions! Limit your total Cheat Fat intake to 1 tablespoon daily. Choose your 1 tablespoon quota from these options:

Butter                     Sour cream

Mayonnaise                 Trans-fat-free margarine

Salad dressings

# SAMPLE CHEAT DAYS

One big key to success on this plan is to eat food you really enjoy 2 days a week. Based on the guidelines above, here's a look at how to put together your cheat days.

| Day 4 |
| --- |

### *Breakfast*

2 scrambled eggs (Smart Protein)
Stack of 3 pancakes (drizzle with sugar-free syrup) (Cheat Carb)
½ grapefruit (Smart Fiber)

### *Snack*

Handful of almonds

### *Lunch*

Lettuce and salad veggies topped with 3 to 4 ounces of chunk light tuna (Smart
  Fiber and Smart Protein), drizzled with 1 tablespoon of olive oil (Smart Fat)
  mixed with 2 tablespoons of balsamic vinegar
1 peach (Smart Carb)

*Snack*

1 medium apple

*Dinner*

Sirloin steak, grilled (Cheat Protein)
Vegetable medley (Smart Fiber)
Tossed salad with 1 tablespoon of salad dressing (Smart Fiber with Cheat Fat)
2 glasses of red wine (Cheat Carb)

## Day 7

*Breakfast*

4 egg whites, scrambled (Smart Protein)
½ cup oatmeal (Smart Carb)
1 fresh pear (Smart Fiber)

*Snack*

Smoothie (see Chapter 5)

*Lunch*

Grilled chicken breast (Smart Protein)
Mashed cauliflower (Smart Fiber)
1 banana (Smart Carb)

*Snack*

Handful of almonds

*Dinner*

Pizza—2 slices, ⅛ to ⅙ of the pie per slice (Cheat Protein and Cheat Carb)
Tossed salad with 1 tablespoon of salad dressing (Smart Fiber with Cheat Fat)
2 light beers (Cheat Carb)

# CHEAT DAYS WORKSHEET

On cheat days, *please write down what you eat at each meal and log in the calorie count.* Doing so will keep you accountable on these days and more aware of the calorie count of your favorite foods. This might sound like a hassle, but it will pay off later and make it easier to keep your weight off in the end!

| Breakfast | Calories |
|---|---|
| My protein: _____ | _____ |
| My fiber: _____ | _____ |
| My carb: _____ | _____ |
| Condiments: _____ | _____ |
| Total calories for breakfast: | _____ |

| Lunch | Calories |
|---|---|
| My protein: _____ | _____ |
| My fiber: _____ | _____ |
| My carb: _____ | _____ |
| Condiments: _____ | _____ |
| Total calories for lunch: | _____ |

| Dinner | Calories |
|--------|----------|

My protein: _____   _____

My fiber: _____   _____

My carb: _____   _____

Condiments: _____   _____

Total calories for dinner:                                _____

| Snacks | Calories |
|--------|----------|

_____   _____

_____   _____

Total calories for snacks:                                _____

**Total daily calories (should not exceed 1,500 for women; 1,800 for men)**                                _____

# CHEATING AT RESTAURANTS

I'm willing to bet that you'll do a lot of your cheating at restaurants. Good idea, as long as you're smart about it. What I like to do is pick one or two temptations, then steer clear of the others. And I'm always in tune with my calorie count on my cheat days. Here are some suggestions:

If you want the pasta (and even then, request a half portion), along with a cocktail or two, ditch the bread and the dessert. Try to stay in control in one way or another. It's like you're bargaining with yourself: *If I don't eat bread, do have salad, and don't have dessert, I'll have two glasses of red wine and a pasta dish.* Sure, this requires a little planning on your part, but a little bit of homework means you *cheat with intention.* No mindlessly scarfing down the bread, ordering drinks, or succumbing to the temptation of dessert—and basically blowing your whole plan.

I eat out a lot, so I've had to be smart about it. Here's what I've learned:

Enjoy an appetizer as your entrée. Go for something that has green, leafy vegetables and is light on sauces. Salad for an entrée is perfect. Request the dressing on the side and use the fork-dip method (dip your fork in the dressing, then spear the salad with the fork). Then enjoy your cocktail, a piece of bread, and, calories permitting, a dessert.

Be portion smart. Restaurant portions tend to be at least double and sometimes triple the standard serving size. So consider sharing an entrée. If you're not sharing, don't think you have to clean your plate. Take the rest to go. Opt for any entrée on the menu that's steamed, grilled, baked, or broiled, and don't even think about ordering anything that is fried or swimming in cheese or cream sauces. And those all-you-can-eat buffets? Forget it, folks. It's just too hard to figure out the calories in all that food, and just too darn tempting. Whenever you're at a restaurant, eat slowly, enjoy your meal, and don't waste your cheat calories on foods that aren't your absolute favorites.

Don't be afraid to go out to eat. Eating out on your cheat days can help you stay on track for success. Why? If you've been eating the same number of calories on your clean days, bumping up that number by 200 to 500 calories one night can increase your metabolism. However, when dining out, be sensible. Don't go crazy to boost the number of calories, since so much restaurant food is loaded with hidden calories. You can eat anything you want and still lose weight, as long as you stay within your caloric parameters.

## THE DRINK SYNC

Diets that ban alcohol entirely are old-style. It is perfectly okay to factor in a drink or two on cheat days. But let me throw up a few red flags here: Alcoholic beverages tend to be high in calories and sugar. Alcohol itself is a carb, and like a lot of carbs, it can cause our bodies to store calories as fat. What's more, alcohol lowers your inhibitions, stimulates your appetite, and leads to all kinds of mindless food transgressions. You just have to be careful, but I've got some ideas for you along those lines.

At restaurants, I recommend the following: Order a strong clear drink, like vodka or tequila, mixed with water or barely a hint of a mixer. For example, instead of a frozen margarita, which can run your calorie tab up as much as 900 calories per drink, order tequila straight up with a splash of margarita mix or lime juice. The intensity and strong flavor of a pure-alcohol drink will cause you to drink it slowly rather than guzzle it down like you would most mixed drinks.

And while I'm on the subject of mixed drinks: Ask for low-calorie or no-calorie mixers, such as seltzer or diet soda. One of the lowest-calorie alcoholic beverages is vodka. For a shot of vodka, you're imbibing only 56 calories per drink versus 116 calories in a regular glass of dry white wine. Plus, you can mix vodka with diet sodas, if you wish. If you're trying to kick the diet soda habit but still prefer something sparkly, request vodka and club soda instead. Don't do tonic water, however; it has almost the same number of calories as a regular soda (150 calories), whereas club soda has zilch. During your meal, drink 8 ounces of water between drinks to stay hydrated and cut back on the number of calories you're swilling.

One more thing, and this is your big brother talking: Never drink and drive, and always drink alcohol responsibly.

## Dolvett's Dos and Don'ts for Cheat Days

*Do* continue to plan your meals according to Dolvett's Dish for breakfast, lunch, and dinner: 1 Smart Protein, 1 Smart Fiber, and 1 Smart Carb at each meal.

*Do* eat at least three meals a day; include snacks, and eat every 2½ to 3 hours.

*Do* understand Cheat Proteins and Cheat Carbs: Substitute or add some of your favorite foods at one of these cheat meals. (See the list below.) For example, for dinner you might have a steak as your Cheat Protein, and add 2 alcoholic beverages, like wine, or a dessert as your Cheat Carb. Or let's say you'd like to cheat at breakfast. Perhaps you'd enjoy a stack of 3 pancakes as your Cheat Carb, along with some scrambled egg whites as your Smart Protein. Is pizza one of your favorite foods? Go ahead and enjoy it! Have 1 or 2 slices of pizza for lunch or dinner as your Cheat Protein and Cheat Carb, maybe with a tossed salad.

*Do* count calories carefully on your cheat days. Don't go above 1,500 calories a day if you're a woman or 1,800 calories a day if you're a man, on your cheat days.

*Do* enjoy everything in moderation. You've heard it from me before, but it's true. A scoop of ice cream isn't going to wreck your waistline, but polishing off the carton will.

*Do* pay attention to portion sizes, and *don't* reach for seconds. Stay away from supersize portions, such as bagels the size of hubcaps and mountain-size platters of pasta.

*Don't* binge, go overboard, or otherwise overindulge. Eat within your calorie limit, and don't overload your stomach.

If you're not hungry, don't eat. Hunger requires a little internal reality check. To see if you're really hungry, *do* know the signals: Your stomach starts to sound like an angry dog, you feel truly empty, and you might even feel shaky (due to low blood sugar). Before grabbing food, drink a glass of water. Sometimes hunger comes masked as thirst.

When you cheat, *do* focus on foods that also provide a nutritional benefit, like dark chocolate, which is full of antioxidants.

For beverages, *do* continue to use distilled water and coconut water. On cheat days, it's fine to drink diet sodas and other sugar-free beverages, but stay within your calorie limits.

*Do* include soups in your daily menus (they are filling) as long as they are broth based. Don't have soups made with milk or cream.

*Do* continue to use condiments in moderation.

*Do* exercise on your cheat days—and work out hard. This will help burn up those extra cheat calories!

*Do* return to clean-day eating after your cheat day.

*Don't* beat yourself up if your cheat becomes a binge or if you have some slipups. It's not possible to gain large amounts of weight from slipups. It's what happens after you overindulge that really counts. Instead of throwing up your hands in defeat, climb back on the healthy wagon right away.

## I DID IT ON DOLVETT'S PROGRAM!

I'm in business for myself, and I often put my health and fitness on hold to focus on building my company. My days were always crammed with business meetings, and I usually worked late, grabbing fast food on the run. I certainly didn't have time to exercise. My weight eventually crept up to 160 pounds. At forty-five years old and at 5'4", that's a lot of heft to carry around. I felt uncomfortable at that weight and was wearing bulky sweaters and jackets—usually in dark colors—to disguise my shape.

I decided to try the 3-1-2-1 Diet because it seemed like it would work well with my lifestyle. Plus, I could do the workout at home early in the morning, or in my office on one of my few breaks. I was amazed that I dropped 15 pounds in just 20 days. I had never experienced that kind of weight loss before. Naturally, the fast weight loss motivated me to keep going, and a few weeks later I reached my goal weight of 130.

My tips:

■ Cook in bulk, especially if you have a busy lifestyle. Cook chicken breasts, brown rice, and veggies ahead of time. Pack them in plastic containers to take to work; this helps you resist the urge to splurge on foods you shouldn't eat.
■ Have smoothies for breakfast. They're quick, convenient, and filling.
■ Memorize restaurant menus. If you eat out a lot like I do, get familiar with the menus of different restaurants. Know what you're going to order ahead of time, and always make the healthiest choices.

—*Veronica C.*

## BETTER CHEAT CHOICES: KEEP HEALTH IN MIND

You can cheat with any food you want, but I'd like you to make choices that will do your body some good. A healthy technique to learn is to pick cheat foods that won't make you fatter or do possible damage to your heart and other organs. Quality food always matters. It's not just a question of cheating for cheating's sake. It's a matter of making better cheat choices. Here are some examples of what I'm talking about:

## Fruit Juice versus Whole Fruit

Yes, you're free to have fruit juice on your cheat days, but it's better to just eat the whole fruit. Because they're devoid of fiber, fruit juices don't take up much space in your stomach, so you'll be left hungry and wanting more food. Fiber-rich fruits, however, help tame your appetite. So whole fruits are always a better choice.

## Milk/Dairy versus Dairy Substitutes

I am not a big fan of cow's milk. Milk may contain added cancer-causing hormones, plus it causes digestive problems for a good part of the population. We're not babies anymore; we don't need milk. What about bone health? Interestingly, the countries with the highest intake of milk have the highest rates of osteoporosis, the bone-thinning disease. You can get bone-building calcium from foods other than milk, such as green vegetables and calcium-fortified dairy substitutes, such as almond milk and coconut milk (my two favorites).

## Mayo versus Mustard

Unless mayo is one of your favorite, must-have cheat foods, use mustard instead. While most brands of mayonnaise have 100 calories in just 1 tablespoon, the average serving of mustard contains barely 3. That's a big difference, obviously. Personally, I prefer mustard over mayo any day.

## Thin-Cut French Fries

French fries are hard to resist. I know, because I love them. But here's where you can enjoy your fries and save on calories too. Trade in regular thin-style fries at 325 calories for a serving of potato wedges or steak fries, 150 calories. You'll save 175 calories.

## Ice Cream Swaps

Two scoops of regular ice cream run around 200 to 300 calories per dish. Choose two scoops of frozen yogurt at 150 calories. Another good strategy is to try some of the reduced-calorie, reduced-fat frozen desserts, such as Fudgsicles or ice cream sandwiches. They are about 150 calories a serving. Better yet, stock up on sugar-free Popsicles at 0 calories a serving.

## Dips That Won't Go to Your Hips

If you're like me, you love dips (the food, not the exercise). Problem is, many will go straight to your hips if you're not careful. Most are loaded with calories, even in a mere tablespoon. Just 2 tablespoons of some dips pack more than 100 calories and more than 10 grams of fat, so calories can stack up fast, especially if you're dipping high-fat chips. A healthier option is to choose salsa or fat-free salad dressings for dipping over other more fattening dips. And dip raw veggies instead of fatty, salty chips.

## Good Chips, Bad Chips

Speaking of chips: As cheat foods, potato and other chips tend to be addictive. The advertising line "I bet you can't eat just one" is so true. As for me, I'd rather spend my cheat calories on something filling, and potato chips don't do it. If you love the crunch of chips, replace fattening potato chips with kale chips, which are available in packages now. Or you can make your own "green" chips: Tear up some kale or collard greens, toss them with a little vegetable spray and Mrs. Dash, and bake them at 300°F for 25 minutes on a cookie sheet until crisp. Check out my recipe for *Spinach Chips* on page 121.

## Salad Dressing Smarts

Salad dressings are allowed on cheat days. But you might want to swap out full-fat dressings for their lighter counterparts. Both types taste basically the same, but with the lighter choice, you could save up to 100 calories.

## The Granola Myth

Here's a cereal that's touted as a health food. But when you consider that ⅔ cup of granola contains 376 calories, lots of sugar, and a fair amount of fat, I don't like granola's résumé. If you like a crunch cereal, go for a bowl of Grape-Nuts at 264 calories in ⅔ cup. That's a savings of 112 calories.

## Stop the Pop

Sure, you can drink soda pop on your cheat days, but why waste the calories? You'll fill up better on solid-food calories. Plus, you're moving toward real lifestyle change (I hope), so maybe it's time to get off the soda habit. Drink fruit-flavored sparkling water instead, or pure water. You'll save around 150 calories every time you quench your thirst with a better, healthier choice.

# HERE'S TO HEALTHY CHOICES

Here's the deal: On your cheat days, focus on eating well for your health, and permanent weight control will continue. Along with cheat foods and cheat meals, include low-calorie, nutritious, natural foods. That means vegetables, fruits, whole grains, and lean proteins. Always seek out better choices in each food category.

Hold yourself to a higher standard and have your diet reflect your good-health consciousness. I believe that eating should be a sensual and enjoyable experience that tantalizes our taste buds, connects us to others, and provides life-enhancing nutrients to our bodies. By selecting carefully and preparing creatively, you can maximize eating pleasure, extend your longevity, and get an amazing body.

## AFFIRM TO GET FIRM: GET OVER THE GUILT

Another good affirmation for this plan is "No food is off-limits." Keep repeating this, because once you accept it as a dietary truth, you won't feel guilty about eating Cheat Proteins or Cheat Carbs. Any behavior that's driven by feelings of guilt is hard to rein in; eating is no exception. Dwelling on slips or overindulgences and regretting your actions does nothing but roadblock your successes.

# 4 The 3-1-2-1 Meal Plans

Planning your meals on the 3-1-2-1 Diet is a cinch. All you need is the right combination of protein, fibers, and carbs in the right proportions and portions at meals to keep your metabolism in fat-burning condition.

When putting together your breakfasts, lunches, and dinners, figure out what your protein, fiber, and carb will be at each meal. Protein should cover about half your plate.

From there, pile on your Smart Fiber. There are many types of Smart Fibers, from vegetables to greens. These foods are so low in calories that you don't have to worry about eating too many of them. However, they should take up at least a fourth of Dolvett's Dish.

Then dish out a Smart Carb. These come in several forms on this diet: fruit carbs, vegetable carbs, and starchy carbs. Choose one type at each main meal. The portion size is 1 piece for fruit carbs, 1 piece or ½ cup (if mashed) for vegetable carbs; and ½ cup (for women) or 1 cup (for men) for starchy carbs. If choosing multigrain bread as one of your starchy carbs, 1 slice of bread equals 1 serving. Basically, your carb serving should take up the remaining part of Dolvett's Dish, after portioning out your Smart Protein and Smart Fiber.

## ADDITIONAL INFO ON CALORIES

As a reminder, on clean days you don't have to obsess too much over your calorie counts, because the proportions and portions on Dolvett's Dish give you the right amount of calories automatically. Even so, I think you ought to have a general awareness of how many calories are in some of the typical foods you'll be eating on both clean days and cheat days. And if you love to do the calorie math, by all means, add up your calories every day and keep track. A good calorie-counting guide can be invaluable. Here are the calorie counts for many of the foods you'll be eating. The counts are approximate and may vary.

### Proteins

Almond milk, 1 cup—60 calories
Beans and legumes, women's portion (½ cup)—100 calories; men's portion
　　(1 cup)—200 calories
*Beef, lean, 4 ounces—207 calories
Coconut milk, 1 cup—50 calories
*Dark meat poultry, skinless, 4 ounces—236 calories
Egg whites, 4 whites—69 calories
Eggs, 2 whole—140 calories
Fattier fish (such as salmon), 4 ounces—233 calories
Greek nonfat yogurt, 1 cup—133 calories
*Lamb, lean, 4 ounces—270 calories
Nonfat cottage cheese, ½ cup—52 calories
*Pork, lean, 4 ounces—237 calories
Protein powders, 1 scoop—50 to 100 calories, depending on product
Shellfish, 4 ounces—112 calories
*Veal, lean, 4 ounces—190 calories
White fish (such as tilapia), 4 ounces—145 calories
White meat chicken, skinless, 4 ounces—186 calories
White meat turkey, skinless, 4 ounces—153 calories

### Fibers

Apple, 1 medium—80 calories
Blackberries, 1 cup—80 calories
Blueberries, 1 cup—82 calories
Broccoli, 1 cup raw—24 calories; 1 cup cooked—46 calories

Grapefruit, ½—50 calories

Green beans, 1 cup cooked—44 calories

Orange, 1 medium—62 calories

Peach, 1 medium—59 calories

Pear, 1 medium—90 calories

Raspberries, 1 cup—61 calories

Salad, lettuce, 1 cup raw—10 calories

Spinach and other greens, 1 cup raw—12 calories; 1 cup cooked—24 calories

Strawberries, 1 cup—45 calories

## Carbs

Banana, 1 medium (7" long)—105 calories

Brown rice, cooked, women's portion (½ cup)—109 calories; men's portion (1 cup)—218 calories

Oatmeal, cooked, women's portion (½ cup)—83 calories; men's portion (1 cup)—166 calories

Parsnips, boiled, 1 medium piece (about 5 inches)—114 calories

*Pasta, preferably whole wheat, women's portion (½ cup)—87 calories; men's portion (1 cup)—174 calories

Quinoa, cooked, women's portion (½ cup)—111 calories; men's portion (1 cup)—222 calories

Sweet potatoes/yams, baked in skin, 1 medium—100 calories

Wild rice, cooked, women's portion (½ cup)—83 calories; men's portion (1 cup)—166 calories

Winter squash, baked, 1 cup—82 calories

## Other

Almonds, 1 handful (¼ cup)—207 calories

Low-fat string cheese, 2 sticks—100 calories

*Foods marked with an asterisk are choices for cheat days.

| My Favorite Fat-Burning Foods | |
|---|---|
| *Food* | *Benefits* |
| Apples | An apple a day makes the fat go away? Maybe. Apples are extremely filling. Try having one before a main meal, and you might eat less. Plus, these luscious fruits are high in fat-fighting fiber. |
| Beans and legumes | These foods are high in protein, which helps burn fat, and are loaded with fiber, which makes you feel full longer. Fiber also ushers unused calories from the body. |
| Cayenne pepper | Cayenne pepper and other spicy foods contain capsaicin, a natural chemical that coaxes the body into producing heat in a process called thermogenesis. This process increases calorie and fat burning. |
| Eggs | Eating eggs at breakfast has been shown in research to curb appetite later in the day and contribute to impressive weight loss. |
| Flaxseed oil | Flaxseed oil promotes fullness and helps trim belly fat. |
| Grapefruit | Natural chemicals in grapefruit lower insulin levels (insulin is a fat-forming hormone) and thus encourage weight loss. The sweet taste of grapefruit can satisfy cravings. |
| Salmon | Salmon is high in omega-3 fatty acids, which support weight loss by normalizing blood sugar and enhancing mood (depression can trigger binge eating). |
| Spinach | Spinach is loaded with magnesium, a mineral that helps the body manufacture serotonin, a feel-good brain chemical. With enough serotonin being produced, you're less likely to feel depressed (depression and obesity are related). |
| Sweet potatoes | Another fiber-rich food, sweet potatoes keep you feeling full longer. They are also digested slowly, especially when eaten with protein. |
| Yogurt | Yogurt is rich in calcium, which can enhance your body's fat-burning mechanisms. |

# MEAL PATTERNS

To get rid of that fat wedged between your muscle and skin, you need every edge possible—which is why meal frequency is superkey to stripping off body fat. One of the reasons the 3-1-2-1 Diet works so well is that you get to eat every 2 to 3 hours. This not only keeps you from getting too hungry and falling off your diet; it also coaxes your body into processing food throughout the day—which keeps your metabolism running in high gear. The net effect is that you'll be eating your way to a lean body.

But before you hit the buffet lines, let me explain this idea of eating your way to leanness. You'll be eating three main meals and two snacks if you're a woman and three to four snacks if you're a man. Your three main meals include quality protein, fiber, and carb sources. For snacks, you'll eat mostly high-fiber foods like almonds, veggies, or fruits; or filling smoothies; or satiating proteins like yogurt or low-fat string cheese sticks. Take a look at the sample menu plans in this chapter, and you'll see what I mean about snacking. It isn't a ton of food, just enough to keep your body fueled and your hunger in check.

Plan those snacks too. To avoid unplanned splurges, don't leave snacking to chance.

Another important issue has to do with timing, particularly around workouts. At breakfast, lunch, and dinner, you'll be eating larger quantities of protein and carbs. Two hours after those meals is a good time to work out because you'll be energized by food.

---

### A Vegetarian-Friendly Plan

People frequently say to me: "I'm a vegetarian. Can I still follow your diet?"
Answer: Yes!

Some people are vegetarians for cultural or personal beliefs or for health reasons. If you prefer to follow a largely plant-based diet, the 3-1-2-1 Diet will work beautifully. If you're the type of vegetarian who can eat some animal-based foods, then enjoy eggs, egg whites, yogurt, cheese, and cottage cheese as some of your proteins. Vegetable proteins such as legumes and lentils are perfect. So are protein powders made with rice or hemp proteins. These are all Smart Proteins; simply substitute them into your menus where protein is called for.

Then, after your workout, have a snack such as a smoothie. At this time, your body is metabolically hungry for protein and carbs. Both nutrients go straight to work, replenishing muscle energy and amino acids depleted during your workouts. This is the perfect way to set your muscle-developing processes in motion.

Then there's the question of when to stop eating for the day. I believe in setting a cutoff time, like not eating 2 to 3 hours prior to bedtime. This allows your body to metabolize food during your waking hours so that it's less likely to be stored away as fat during sleep.

## CHEAT SHEET!

Like your clean meals and snacks, you'll want to plan your cheat days so that they don't turn into total food orgies. The sample cheat days I've got for you provide similar amounts of protein, carbs, and fat as your typical clean days, though you can toss in some you've been craving, like pizza. Most of your extra calories on cheat days will probably come from carbohydrates, such as pasta, potatoes, breads, a cocktail or two, and desserts.

This bears repeating: Having cheat days keeps your metabolism guessing, as opposed to letting it get used to one particular caloric level day after day, and this keeps your fat-burning engines revving. Just as you need to change things up in your workouts for continued body-shaping progress, you must vary your diet so your body doesn't get used to the same foods day after day. This is why I've planned this diet to give you cheat days. It's all about shocking the metabolism into action.

## THE MEAL PLANS

I suggest that you begin my 3-1-2-1 Diet like this: Follow these meals plans, week by week. They'll give you structure, and there's no guesswork—all of which helps guard again unplanned eating. Also, you can learn about foods and new ways to prepare them, with the help of my recipes in the next chapter.

If you need more food flexibility, feel free to change the order of the menus or use the menus you like as often as you want. (Just leave the cheat days in day 4 and day 7 of each week.) It's okay to substitute foods with others in the same food group too. For example, if you can't stomach fish, substitute chicken or another protein. Just don't skimp on foods or try to drastically cut back your calories. You'll only feel deprived, and that's not what this diet is about. Be creative with your snacks and make good choices to satisfy your taste buds.

# MY 21-DAY MENU PLAN

## Day 1

### Breakfast

4 scrambled egg whites (1 Smart Protein)
1 tomato, sliced (1 Smart Fiber)
1 medium banana (7" long) (1 Smart Carb)

### Snack

Handful of almonds (¼ cup)

### Lunch

*Chicken Almond Salad*, page 110 (1 Smart Protein and 1 Smart Fiber)
1 cup of chopped fresh pineapple (1 Smart Carb)

### Snack

*A+ Smoothie*, page 105

### Dinner

About 4 ounces of grilled salmon (1 Smart Protein)
1 cup of steamed broccoli (1 Smart Fiber)
1 baked sweet potato, medium (1 Smart Carb)

*Men: Add 2 extra snacks: ¼ cup of almonds and 1 medium banana.*

*Total Calories/Women: 1,200*
*Total Calories/Men: 1,565*

## Day 2

### Breakfast

*Rise and Grind Smoothie*, page 104 (1 Smart Protein, 1 Smart Fiber, and 1 Smart Carb)

### Snack

1 medium apple

### Lunch

*Ranch Lettuce Wraps*, page 110 (1 Smart Protein and 1 Smart Fiber)
½ cup of cooked quinoa for women; 1 cup for men (1 Smart Carb)

### Snack

2 sticks of low-fat string cheese

### Dinner

*Easy Roast Turkey*, page 117 (1 Smart Protein)
1 cup of steamed green beans (1 Smart Fiber)
½ cup of cooked brown rice for women; 1 cup for men (1 Smart Carb)

*Men: Add an extra snack of 1 handful (¼ cup) of almonds.*

*Total Calories/Women: 1,145*
*Total Calories/Men: 1,572*

## Day 3

*Breakfast*

*Veggie Omelet*, page 107 (1 Smart Protein and 1 Smart Fiber)
½ cup of cooked oatmeal for women; 1 cup for men (1 Smart Carb)

*Snack*

*Yogurt Berry Shake*, page 105 (1 Smart Protein, 1 Smart Carb, and
    1 Smart Fiber)

*Lunch*

Shrimp cocktail: Fresh boiled or thawed-from-frozen shrimp (about 4 ounces)
    (1 Smart Protein) with 2 tablespoons of cocktail sauce made from reduced-
    sugar ketchup mixed with horseradish
½ cup of sliced cucumber drizzled with 1 tablespoon of olive oil + 1 tablespoon of
    white vinegar, seasoned with Mrs. Dash (1 Smart Fiber)
1 medium peach (1 Smart Carb)

*Snack*

1 serving of *Spinach Chips*, page 121 (1 Smart Fiber)

*Dinner*

2 lean ground turkey patties (about 3 ounces each) (1 Smart Protein)
1 cup of stewed tomatoes (1 Smart Fiber)
½ cup of cooked brown rice for women; 1 cup for men (1 Smart Carb)

*Men: Add 1 medium apple as an extra snack.*

*Total Calories/Women: 1,231*
*Total Calories/Men: 1,503*

## Day 4 (Cheat Day)

### Breakfast

2 scrambled egg whites (1 Smart Protein)

1 slice of multigrain gluten-free bread for women; 2 slices for men
    (1 Smart Carb)

1 cup of sliced strawberries (1 Smart Fiber)

### Snack

1 medium orange

### Lunch

1 slice of pizza (⅙ to ⅛ pie) for women; 2 slices for men
    (1 Cheat Carb and 1 Cheat Protein)

Tossed salad with 2 tablespoons of salad dressing
    (1 Smart Fiber and 1 Cheat Fat)

### Snack

1 medium pear

### Dinner

Sirloin steak (1 Cheat Protein)

Baked potato with sour cream or butter (1 Cheat Carb, 1 Cheat Fat)

Vegetable medley (1 Smart Fiber)

2 glasses of red wine (1 Cheat Carb)

*Total Calories/Women: 1,509*
*Total Calories/Men: 1,859*

## Day 5

### Breakfast

1 hard-boiled egg (½ Smart Protein)

½ cup of cooked oatmeal with ½ cup of almond milk for women;
   1 cup of cooked oatmeal with 1 cup of almond milk for men
   (1 Smart Carb with ½ Smart Protein)

1 fresh pear, sliced (1 Smart Fiber)

### Snack

*Yogurt Berry Shake*, page 105 (1 Smart Protein, 1 Smart Carb, and
   1 Smart Fiber)

### Lunch

Open-faced turkey sandwich: 1 slice multigrain gluten-free bread (1 Smart Carb)
   topped with 4 slices of fat-free turkey ham (1 Smart Protein); spread bread
   with dark mustard, if desired

1 cup of grape or cherry tomatoes (1 Smart Fiber)

### Snack

Handful of almonds (¼ cup)

### Dinner

*Vegetarian-Style Chili*, page 113 (1 Smart Protein, 1 Smart Carb, and
   1 Smart Fiber)

*Men: Add 1 medium apple as an extra snack.*

*Total Calories/Women: 1,201*
*Total Calories/Men: 1,503*

## Day 6

*Breakfast*

*Peachy Keen Shake*, page 106 (1 Smart Protein, 1 Smart Fiber, and 1 Smart Carb)

*Snack*

1 medium orange

*Lunch*

*Spinach Salad*, page 111 (1 Smart Protein and 1 Smart Fiber)
½ of a cantaloupe (1 Smart Carb)

*Snack*

1 serving of *Spinach Chips*, page 121 (1 Smart Fiber)

*Dinner*

*Oriental Chicken with Hot Garlic Sauce*, page 116 (1 Smart Protein and
   1 Smart Fiber)
Serve over ½ cup brown rice for women; 1 cup for men (1 Smart Carb)

*Men: Add 1 extra serving of* Spinach Chips, *page 121, and ¼ cup of almonds.*

*Total Calories/Women: 1,231*
*Total Calories/Men: 1,531*

## Day 7 (Cheat Day)

*Breakfast*

2 pancakes (any type, 6" diameter) for women; 4 pancakes for men, drizzled with
   sugar-free maple syrup (1 Cheat Carb)

2 slices of bacon (have turkey bacon if you are watching your cholesterol)
    (1 Cheat Protein)
1 cup of blueberries (1 Smart Fiber)

### Snack

1 medium pear

### Lunch

*Chicken Cobb Salad*, page 109 (1 Smart Protein and 1 Smart Fiber)
1 medium orange (1 Smart Carb)

### Dinner

*Dinner at a Mexican restaurant:*
1 jigger (1½ ounces) of tequila, mixed with water or sugar-free margarita mix
    (Cheat Carb)
2 beef fajitas in 2 (8") tortillas (flour) (1 Cheat Protein and 1 Cheat Carb),
    topped with salsa
½ cup of pico de gallo (1 Smart Fiber)

---

### Restaurant Calorie Red Alert!

A Mexican dinner like this can add up to 500 calories or more, depending on the restaurant. Be familiar with meal calories at restaurants before you go.

---

*Men: Add 1 medium banana as an extra snack.*

---

*Total Calories/Women: 1,483*
*Total Calories/Men: 1,886*

## Day 8

*Breakfast*

2 scrambled eggs (1 Smart Protein)
1 cup of sliced fresh strawberries (1 Smart Fiber)
½ cup of cooked oatmeal for women; 1 cup for men (1 Smart Carb)

*Snack*

1 medium banana (7" long)

*Lunch*

*Vegetable Bean Salad*, page 112, ½ cup for women; 1 cup for men (1 Smart
    Protein and 1 Smart Fiber)
1 slice of multigrain gluten-free bread for women; 2 slices for men (1 Smart Carb)

*Snack*

*Yogurt Berry Shake*, page 105 (1 Smart Protein, 1 Smart Carb, and 1 Smart Fiber)

*Dinner*

*Easy Roast Turkey*, page 117 (1 Smart Protein)
½ cup of *Maple Orange Mashed Sweet Potatoes*, page 122 (1 Smart Carb)
1 cup of steamed green beans (1 Smart Fiber)

---

*Total Calories/Women: 1,238*
*Total Calories/Men: 1,567*

## Day 9

*Breakfast*

*Tropical Delight* smoothie, page 104 (1 Smart Protein, 1 Smart Carb, and
    1 Smart Fiber)

*Snack*

2 sticks of low-fat string cheese

*Lunch*

*Chicken Cobb Salad*, page 109 (1 Smart Protein and 1 Smart Fiber)
1 medium peach (1 Smart Carb)

*Snack*

1 cup of fresh strawberries, topped with 1 tablespoon of nonfat Greek yogurt

*Dinner*

*Vegetarian-Style Chili*, page 113 (1 Smart Protein, 1 Smart Carb, and
    1 Smart Fiber)
Tossed side salad drizzled with 1 tablespoon of olive oil and 2 tablespoons of
    balsamic vinegar (1 Smart Fiber and 1 optional Smart Fat)

*Men: Add an extra snack of 1 cup of sliced strawberries with 1 tablespoon of nonfat
Greek yogurt.*

*Total Calories/Women: 1,223*
*Total Calories/Men: 1,482*

## Day 10

*Breakfast*

*Italian Frittata*, page 107 (1 Smart Protein and 1 Smart Fiber)
1 slice of multigrain, gluten-free toast for women; 2 slices for men
    (1 Smart Carb)

*Snack*

*Rise and Grind Smoothie*, page 104 (1 Smart Protein, 1 Smart Carb, and
    1 Smart Fiber)

*Lunch*

*Taco-Less Salad*, page 114 (1 Smart Protein and 1 Smart Fiber)
1 medium apple (1 Smart Carb)

*Snack*

1 cup of raw, cut-up veggies and 2 sticks of low-fat string cheese

*Dinner*

Grilled chicken breast (about 4 ounces) (1 Smart Protein)
*Dolvett's Mock Mashed Potatoes*, page 123 (1 Smart Fiber and
    1 Smart Carb)

*Men: Add ¼ cup of almonds as an extra snack.*

**Total Calories/Women: 1,251**
**Total Calories/Men: 1,536**

## Day 11 (Cheat Day)

### Breakfast

*Rise and Grind Smoothie*, page 104 (1 Smart Protein, 1 Smart Carb, and
    1 Smart Fiber)

### Snack

1 medium apple

### Lunch

Cheeseburger with a whole-grain bun (1 Cheat Protein and 1 Cheat Carb) with
    lettuce and tomato (1 Smart Fiber)

### Snack

Skinny Cow ice cream sandwich

### Dinner

2 lamb chops (1 Cheat Protein)
*Sweet Potato Fries*, page 123 (1 Smart Carb)
1 cup of steamed asparagus (1 Smart Fiber)

*Men: Add the* A+ Smoothie, *page 105, as an extra snack.*

*Total Calories/Women: 1,447*
*Total Calories/Men: 1,756*

## Day 12

*Breakfast*

*Fruity Breakfast Salad*, page 109 (1 Smart Protein, 1 Smart Carb, and
1 Smart Fiber)

*Snack*

1 serving of *Spinach Chips*, page 121

*Lunch*

Baked or broiled chicken breast (about 5 ounces) (1 Smart Protein)
*Quinoa Apple Salad*, page 120 (1 Smart Carb and 1 Smart Fiber)

*Snack*

Large bowl of *Veggistrone*, page 124

*Dinner*

*Zucchini Lasagna*, page 115 (1 Smart Protein and 1 Smart Fiber)
1 cup of chopped fresh pineapple (1 Smart Carb)

*Men: Add* Tropical Delight *smoothie, page 104, as an extra snack.*

*Total Calories/Women: 1,224*
*Total Calories/Men: 1,510*

## Day 13

*Breakfast*

A+ *Smoothie*, page 105 (1 Smart Protein, 1 Smart Fiber, and
    1 Smart Carb)

*Snack*

1 cup of raspberries

*Lunch*

*Smart Tuna Salad*, page 112 (1 Smart Protein and 1 Smart Fiber)
1 cup of chopped pineapple (1 Smart Carb)

*Snack*

1 cup of nonfat Greek yogurt sweetened with Truvia

*Dinner*

*Oriental Chicken with Hot Garlic Sauce*, page 116 (1 Smart Protein and
    1 Smart Fiber)
Serve over ½ cup brown rice for women; 1 cup for men (1 Smart Carb)

*Men: Add a handful of almonds (¼ cup) as an extra snack.*

*Total Calories/Women: 1,255*
*Total Calories/Men: 1,462*

## Day 14 (Cheat Day)

*Breakfast*

2 slices Canadian bacon (1 Smart Protein)

1 waffle (any type, 6" square) for women; 2 waffles for men, drizzled with sugar-
  free maple syrup (1 Cheat Carb)

1 cup of sliced strawberries (1 Smart Fiber)

*Snack*

1 serving of *Spinach Chips*, page 121

*Lunch*

Large bowl of *Veggistrone*, page 124 (1 Smart Fiber)

Grilled cheese sandwich made with 2 slices of bread (any type, although multigrain
  bread is the best choice) and 2 slices of American cheese (1 Cheat Carb and
  1 Cheat Protein)

*Snack*

1 medium apple

*Dinner*

*Dinner at a barbecue restaurant:*

Barbecued beef or pork (about 1 cup) (1 Cheat Protein)

½ cup of creamy or vinegar-based coleslaw (1 Smart Fiber and 1 Cheat Fat)

1 dinner roll (2" square by 2" high) (1 Cheat Carb)

1 light beer (1 Cheat Carb)

---

### Restaurant Calorie Red Alert!

A barbecue dinner like this can add up to 640 calories or more, depending on the restaurant. Be familiar with meal calories at restaurants before you go.

---

*Men: Add a* Yogurt Berry Shake, *page 105, as an extra snack.*

---

*Total Calories/Women: 1,482*
*Total Calories/Men: 1,836*

## Day 15

*Breakfast*

*Biggest Winner French Toast*, page 108: 1 slice for women; 2 slices for men
    (1 Smart Protein and 1 Smart Carb)
1 cup of fresh berries (any type) (1 Smart Fiber)

*Snack*

1 medium peach

*Lunch*

2 ground turkey patties (about 3 ounces each), cooked (1 Smart Protein)
1 sliced tomato (1 Smart Fiber)
*Sweet Potato Fries*, page 123 (1 Smart Carb)

*Snack*

*Tropical Delight* smoothie, page 104

### Dinner

*Stuffed Salmon*, page 117 (1 Smart Protein and 1 Smart Carb)
1 cup of steamed broccoli (1 Smart Fiber)

*Men: Add 1 handful (¼ cup) of almonds as an extra snack.*

> *Total Calories/Women: 1,152*
> *Total Calories/Men: 1,479*

## Day 16

### Breakfast

*Veggie Omelet*, page 107 (1 Smart Protein and 1 Smart Fiber)
1 medium banana (7" long) (1 Smart Carb)

### Snack

*Yogurt Berry Shake*, page 105

### Lunch

*Chicken Almond Salad*, page 110 (1 Smart Protein and 1 Smart Fiber)
1 medium peach

### Snack

2 sticks of low-fat string cheese

### Dinner

*Lean and Tasty Meatloaf*, page 118 (1 Smart Protein and 1 Smart Carb)
1 cup of steamed spinach (1 Smart Fiber)

*Men: Add the* A+ Smoothie, *page 105, as an extra snack.*

Total Calories/Women: 1,208
Total Calories/Men: 1,507

## Day 17

### Breakfast

4 scrambled egg whites (1 Smart Protein)
1 tomato, sliced (1 Smart Fiber)
1 medium banana (7" long) (1 Smart Carb)

### Snack

1 serving of *Spinach Chips*, page 121

### Lunch

Baked or broiled chicken breast (about 4 ounces) (1 Smart Protein)
*Quinoa Apple Salad*, page 120 (1 Smart Carb and 1 Smart Fiber)

### Snack

*Rise and Grind Smoothie*, page 104

### Dinner

*Sweet and Sour Shrimp*, page 119, with *"Fried" Rice*, page 121
    (1 Smart Protein, 1 Smart Fiber, and 1 Smart Carb)

*Men: Add a handful of almonds (¼ cup) and 2 sticks of low-fat string cheese as extra snacks.*

Total Calories/Women: 1,252
Total Calories/Men: 1,559

## Day 18 (Cheat Day)

*Breakfast*

*Veggie Omelet*, page 107 (1 Smart Protein and 1 Smart Fiber)
½ cup of cooked oatmeal for women; 1 cup for men (1 Smart Carb)

*Snack*

Handful of almonds (¼ cup)

*Lunch*

*Lunch at a deli restaurant:*
Pastrami or other deli meat (2 slices) and Swiss cheese (1 slice) on rye bread
   (2 slices) with dark mustard and lettuce and tomato (1 Cheat Protein,
   1 Cheat Carb, and 1 Smart Fiber)

### Restaurant Calorie Red Alert!

A deli lunch like this can add up to 450 calories or more, depending on the deli. Cut calories when ordering by asking for mustard instead of mayo.

*Snack*

1 medium apple

*Dinner*

Pot roast (1 Cheat Protein)
Roasted potato, cut in chunks (1 Cheat Carb)
Cooked vegetables (1 Smart Carb)
1 slice of cheesecake (⅙ of the cake) for dessert (1 Cheat Carb)

*Men: Add the* A+ Smoothie, *page 105, as an extra snack.*

**Total Calories/Women: 1,499**
**Total Calories/Men: 1,808**

## Day 19

### Breakfast

*Rise and Grind Smoothie*, page 104 (1 Smart Protein, 1 Smart Fiber, and
    1 Smart Carb)

### Snack

1 medium pear

### Lunch

Baked or grilled chicken breast (about 4 ounces) (1 Smart Protein)
*Veggistrone*, page 124 (1 Smart Fiber)
1 medium peach (1 Smart Carb)

### Snack

*Yogurt Berry Shake*, page 105

### Dinner

*Easy Roast Turkey*, page 117 (1 Smart Protein)
½ cup of *Maple Orange Mashed Sweet Potatoes*, page 122 (1 Smart Carb)
1 cup of steamed green beans (1 Smart Fiber)

*Men: Add a handful (¼ cup) of almonds and 1 medium banana (7" long) as extra snacks.*

**Total Calories/Women: 1,150**
**Total Calories/Men: 1,462**

## Day 20

*Breakfast*

2 scrambled eggs (1 Smart Protein)
1 cup sliced fresh strawberries (1 Smart Fiber)
½ cup of oatmeal for women; 1 cup of oatmeal for men (1 Smart Carb)

*Snack*

1 medium pear

*Lunch*

*Smart Tuna Salad*, page 112 (1 Smart Protein and 1 Smart Fiber)
1 medium peach (1 Smart Carb)

*Snack*

*Yogurt Berry Shake*, page 105

*Dinner*

Grilled or baked tilapia (about 4 ounces) (1 Smart Protein)
1 cup of baked acorn squash (1 Smart Carb)
1 cup of steamed broccoli or other green vegetable (1 Smart Fiber)

*Men: Add an* A+ Smoothie, *page 105, as an extra snack.*

*Total Calories/Women: 1,165*
*Total Calories/Men: 1,557*

## Day 21 (Cheat Day)

*Breakfast*

1 medium bagel (any type, although whole-grain is the healthier choice),
   3½" diameter (1 Cheat Carb) with 1 tablespoon of reduced-fat
   cream cheese
1 cup of nonfat Greek yogurt (1 Smart Protein)
1 cup of fresh berries, any type (1 Smart Fiber)

*Snack*

Handful (¼ cup) of almonds

*Lunch*

*Vegetarian-Style Chili*, page 113 (1 Smart Protein, 1 Smart Carb, and
   1 Smart Fiber)

*Snack*

1 medium apple

*Dinner*

*Dinner at an Asian restaurant:*
Egg-drop soup, 1 cup
Moo goo gai pan (1 Smart Protein and 1 Smart Fiber)
½ cup steamed brown rice for women; 1 cup for men (1 Smart Carb)

### Restaurant Calorie Red Alert!

An Asian dinner like this can add up to 500 calories
or more, depending on the restaurant. Sweet and
sour and fried entrées will always be higher in
calories than most meat and veggie dishes, so make
smart choices, even on your cheat days.

*Total Calories/Women: 1,572*
*Total Calories/Men: 1,790*

# SMART SHOPPING

Plan your week out based on the above menus. Check your pantry and fridge for foods you need and put them on your shopping list. You may be cooking for your family, so judge how much of each food you'll need to prepare meals. Many fruits and vegetables are seasonal; it's okay to substitute any fruit or vegetable for another if you can't find produce that's in season. If you find you're not going to use fresh proteins within a day or two after purchasing them, be sure to freeze them.

Make sure, too, that you have enough of the following condiments, spices, seasonings, and other staples on hand for food preparation:

Balsamic vinegar

Bay leaves

Chicken broth, fat-free

Chili powder

Cinnamon

Cream cheese, reduced-fat

Garlic powder

Ginger, powdered

Honey

Horseradish

Hot sauce

Ketchup, reduced-sugar

Maple syrup, sugar-free

Mrs. Dash

Mustard

Mustard, ground

Nutmeg

Olive oil

Orange marmalade, sugar-free

Oregano, dried

Parmesan cheese, fat-free

Pepper

Poultry seasoning

Pumpkin pie spice

Raspberry vinegar

Red pepper flakes

Red wine vinegar

Relish, unsweetened

Sage leaves, dried

Salad dressing, light

Salsa

Sesame seeds

Soy sauce, lite (reduced-sodium)

Taco seasoning

Thyme, dried                    White vinegar
Truvia                          Worcestershire sauce
Vegetable cooking spray

---

## Dolvett's Dos and Don'ts for Grocery Shopping

*Do* stick to your shopping list.

*Don't* shop when you're hungry. You might be tempted to buy diet-blowing foods that you don't need.

*Do* use visual cues to select the leanest cuts of meat. Inspect the meat and note how much white is present. The white is nasty, saturated fat. Then check the cut of meat. Select items with "loin" or "round" in the name, such as tenderloin or ground round. They're less fatty.

*Do* shop seasonally for produce. This guarantees you're getting the highest quality and best nutrition for your buck. (Seasonal fruits and veggies are often cheaper than out-of-season produce.)

*Do* read labels to identify added sugar in foods. When I'm shopping, I always read labels. I steer clear of foods with high-fructose corn syrup in them. Since the 1970s, we've been eating gobs of this additive, which is used to sweeten soda, commercial baked goods, and even condiments. If you looked at a chart depicting our nation's rise in obesity and a chart depicting a rise in our consumption of high-fructose corn syrup, you'd see that the two charts parallel each other. It's like the more high-fructose corn syrup we eat, the fatter we get as a country. It's not always easy to determine whether foods contain added sugars, though. Sugar comes in various disguises: dextrose, lactose, evaporated cane juice, molasses, barley malt syrup, and anything that includes the word "sugar" or "syrup" is sugar.

*Do* check the calories per serving. When one serving of a single food item has more than 400 calories per serving, it is loaded with calories.

*Do* shop the perimeter of the store mostly. This is generally where the healthiest and freshest foods reside.

## Week 1 Shopping List

| Vegetables | Quantity needed |
|---|---|
| ❏ Broccoli | |
| ❏ Carrots | |
| ❏ Celery | |
| ❏ Cherry or grape tomatoes | |
| ❏ Cucumbers | |
| ❏ Green beans | |
| ❏ Green onions | |
| ❏ Lettuce | |
| ❏ Onions | |
| ❏ Spinach | |
| ❏ Sweet potatoes | |
| ❏ Tomatoes | |

| Fruits | Quantity needed |
|---|---|
| ❏ Apples | |
| ❏ Bananas | |
| ❏ Blueberries or other berries in season | |
| ❏ Oranges | |
| ❏ Peaches | |
| ❏ Pears | |
| ❏ Pineapple | |
| ❏ Strawberries | |

| Proteins | Quantity needed |
|---|---|
| ❏ Almond milk | |
| ❏ Cartons of eggs | |
| ❏ Chicken breasts | |
| ❏ Coconut milk | |
| ❏ Greek nonfat yogurt | |
| ❏ Salmon fillets | |
| ❏ Shrimp | |
| ❏ Turkey breasts | |
| ❏ Turkey ham, nonfat | |

| Nonperishables | Quantity needed |
|---|---|
| ❏ Canned kidney beans | |
| ❏ Canned pumpkin | |
| ❏ Canned stewed tomatoes | |

| Frozen Foods | Quantity needed |
|---|---|
| ❏ Broccoli florets | |
| ❏ Blueberries | |
| ❏ Peaches | |
| ❏ Toaster pancakes | |

| Grains | Quantity needed |
|---|---|
| ❏ Brown rice | |
| ❏ Multigrain gluten-free bread | |
| ❏ Oatmeal | |
| ❏ Quinoa | |

| Snacks | Quantity needed |
|---|---|
| ❏ Almonds, raw | |

# Week 2 Shopping List

| Vegetables | Quantity needed |
|---|---|
| ❑ Asparagus | |
| ❑ Basil, fresh | |
| ❑ Bell pepper, green | |
| ❑ Bell pepper, red | |
| ❑ Cabbage | |
| ❑ Cauliflower | |
| ❑ Garlic | |
| ❑ Green beans | |
| ❑ Lettuce | |
| ❑ Onion, red | |
| ❑ Spinach | |
| ❑ Sweet potatoes | |
| ❑ Tomatoes | |
| ❑ Zucchini | |

| Fruits | Quantity needed |
|---|---|
| ❑ Apples | |
| ❑ Bananas | |
| ❑ Blueberries | |
| ❑ Pineapple | |
| ❑ Raspberries | |
| ❑ Strawberries | |

| Proteins | Quantity needed |
|---|---|
| ❑ American cheese slices | |
| ❑ Canadian bacon | |
| ❑ Cartons of eggs | |
| ❑ Cottage cheese, nonfat | |
| ❑ Greek nonfat yogurt | |
| ❑ Lamb chops | |
| ❑ Tuna, chunk light, canned | |
| ❑ Turkey breasts | |
| ❑ Turkey, lean, ground | |

| Nonperishables | Quantity needed |
|---|---|
| ❑ Canned diced tomatoes | |
| ❑ Canned garbanzo beans | |
| ❑ Canned kidney beans | |
| ❑ Canned pumpkin | |
| ❑ Canned stewed tomatoes | |
| ❑ Tomato sauce | |

| Frozen Foods | Quantity needed |
|---|---|
| ❑ Toaster waffles | |

| Grains | Quantity needed |
|---|---|
| ❑ Multigrain gluten-free bread | |

| Snacks | Quantity needed |
|---|---|
| ❑ Almonds, raw | |
| ❑ Low-fat string cheese | |
| ❑ Skinny Cow ice cream sandwiches | |

## Week 3 Shopping List

| Vegetables | Quantity needed |
|---|---|
| ❑ Acorn squash | |
| ❑ Bell pepper, green | |
| ❑ Bell pepper, red | |
| ❑ Broccoli | |
| ❑ Lettuce | |
| ❑ Onions | |
| ❑ Potatoes, white | |
| ❑ Spinach | |
| ❑ Sweet potatoes | |
| ❑ Tomatoes | |

| Fruits | Quantity needed |
|---|---|
| ❑ Apples | |
| ❑ Bananas | |
| ❑ Blueberries or other berries in season | |
| ❑ Peaches | |
| ❑ Pears | |
| ❑ Strawberries | |

| Proteins | Quantity needed |
|---|---|
| ❑ Almond milk | |
| ❑ Cartons of eggs | |
| ❑ Chicken breasts | |
| ❑ Coconut milk | |
| ❑ Greek nonfat yogurt | |
| ❑ Pot roast | |
| ❑ Salmon fillets | |
| ❑ Shrimp | |
| ❑ Tilapia fillets | |
| ❑ Tuna, chunk light, canned | |
| ❑ Turkey breasts | |
| ❑ Turkey, lean ground | |

| Nonperishables | Quantity needed |
|---|---|
| ❑ Canned kidney beans | |

| Frozen Foods | Quantity needed |
|---|---|
| ❑ Blueberries or other berries | |
| ❑ Cheesecake | |

| Grains | Quantity needed |
|---|---|
| ❑ Bagels, 6" diameter | |
| ❑ Multigrain gluten-free bread | |

| Snacks | Quantity needed |
|---|---|
| ❑ Almonds, raw | |
| ❑ Almonds, slivered | |
| ❑ Low-fat string cheese | |

# NEXT STEPS

You've now got 3 weeks of sample menus to follow. Now's a good time to take some measurements, especially at your waist, hips, and thighs, and check your weight. Write down this information. Stick it up where you'll see it often, to stay motivated and keep losing. From this point forward, follow these menus over the upcoming weeks, or plan your own meals using the guidelines of my 3-1-2-1 Diet. Your body will keep changing for the better—and so will your life. Congratulations!

# 5 The Key Is in the Kitchen

Where's the most important place for weight loss? If you answered "the gym," you're wrong. It's the kitchen! In this room is where healthy choices really begin. If you get the kitchen right, you get your life right.

If you don't do much cooking, however, learn some basics. It will definitely be good for your waistline as well as your wallet. When you learn to cook or cook more often at home, you have complete control over what goes in your mouth, not to mention the size of your portions.

What I've got for you here is a bumper crop of more than thirty delicious recipes designed to fit into the 3-1-2-1 Diet. They're easy to make and hassle-free, and some can even be frozen for later. Make it a point to try at least a few of these recipes each week. They'll help you make good choices, and when you do that, you'll be successful.

## TIME-SAVERS

I realize, too, that you might be ultrabusy. I know, because I am. So before we start rattling those pots and pans, let me give you a few shortcuts:

- Stock up on frozen ready-to-go veggies. That way you don't have to do any washing, cutting, or chopping—or worry that fresh vegetables will go bad in the fridge. Plus, you can toss shrimp or chicken into frozen stir-fry vegetables, cook, and season with some lite soy sauce. Serve them with some cooked brown rice on the side, and you've just made the perfect Dolvett's Dish for dinner.

- Fix a big pot of healthy soup or chili and freeze the leftovers in single-serve containers.
- Buy precut and bagged lettuce for salads, and frozen unsweetened fruit for smoothies.
- Keep pop-top tuna or salmon cans around. They're portable, and you don't need a can opener.
- Purchase cooked, bagged chicken breasts in the market's meat or deli section. These products are superconvenient and handy for preparing meals and salads.
- Buy prepared vegetable trays and keep them readily available for snacks.
- Buy precooked shrimp for a quick seafood meal.
- For healthy fast-food breakfasts, whip up one of my smoothies (see the recipes later in this chapter). If you've got the right ingredients on hand, these breakfasts in a glass take just minutes to make.

## KITCHEN GEAR

Cooking skillfully is a lot like working out: You've got to have the right gear. I've whipped up a list of kitchen essentials for both new and experienced cooks. For this diet and its recipes, make sure you have the following on hand:

- Baking dishes, 9"
- Blender or food processor
- Colander and sieve
- Cutting boards
- Food scale
- Grater
- Hand mixer
- Large sauté pan or skillet
- Large soup pot
- Loaf pan
- Measuring cups and spoons
- Pie pan, 9"

- Saucepan
- Set of good cutting knives
- Small sauté pan or skillet
- Spatula

## I DID IT ON DOLVETT'S PROGRAM!

For a dieter, I have the worst job in the world: I'm a chef! I'm around food all day, and it is very tempting, as you might imagine. As a result, I hadn't paid much attention to my body. I was soft and fluffy like the lemon meringue pies I baked for customers.

I was really attracted to the concept of cheat days on this diet. I felt like they gave me some leeway. I could splurge and not deprive myself of the foods I love and love to cook. The diet seemed perfect for someone in my profession.

Before, I hadn't worked out much (that's why I looked like a pie!), so the exercise part was new to me. It made sense: a combo of weight training and aerobics all in one. And I enjoyed it. After about a month, I could see some biceps, triceps, and quads under my skin, so obviously I was gaining muscle and losing fat. I dropped about 15 pounds. And with all the food I got to eat, I've even started developing my own recipes that my family and I can eat and enjoy. It's not so bad being a chef after all!

My tips:

- Get back on the wagon. If I overdo it (too many cheats), I don't wait until Monday to restart the plan; I get back on track the very next meal.
- Don't like to cook? Forget about it—everyone can cook something. Try some easy recipes at first. People who cook at home and eat at home can control their food better because they can cook with healthy ingredients. Restaurant food often has hidden fat and sugar in it. I should know because I'm in the restaurant business!
- Modify your favorite recipes. Just about any recipe can be downsized in terms of calories, sugar, and fat. Replace sugar with Truvía, fat with pureed fruit, cream with yogurt—the list goes on. Have fun when you experiment!

*—Jordan T.*

# THE 3-1-2-1 DIET RECIPES

As part of taking off pounds, I encourage you to try several of my recipes each week. Learning new dishes, in addition to reinventing existing ones (see my tips on page 125), is a great strategy for success. Among the most compelling feedback I get from my clients, as well as my *Biggest Loser* team, is how amazed they are that they're not ravenous all the time. They come to the ranch, for example, expecting to be in painful hunger because they're so used to that dieting and deprivation. But with recipes like the ones in this chapter, very seldom do they feel hungry.

Each recipe provides its calorie count, plus how to count it in your diet as a Smart Protein, Smart Fiber, Smart Carb, or combination dish.

Here's a key to help you find each one of these delicious dishes:

### *Smoothies*

### *Breakfasts*

### *Lunches*

# SMOOTHIES FOR BREAKFAST AND SNACKS

For a meal that's supposed to be the most important of the day, breakfast sure doesn't rate too high. A single cup of coffee or a doughnut or two at work is as much as many people take time for. Folks, I've got a better idea, and it doesn't involve getting up at the crack of dawn: smoothies. Just toss some frozen fruit and yogurt or nut milk into a blender, and you're good to go. (I also add oats, veggies, or protein powder for more substance.) If you've got some seriously ripe fruit (like a banana) that's limping around, don't put it down the garbage disposal! Just cover it with foil and throw it in the freezer.

You'll have quick and healthy ingredients for your smoothies. Sweeten your smoothie according to your preferences. I like honey in my smoothies, though using Truvía instead cuts calories significantly. Smoothies make great pre-workout or post-workout snacks too.

## Rise and Grind Smoothie

*INGREDIENTS*

   1 cup of almond milk

   ½ cup of frozen unsweetened berries

   Handful of fresh spinach

   1 tablespoon of honey or 1 to 2 packets of Truvía

*PREPARATION*

Place all ingredients in a blender and puree until smooth.

*Makes 1 serving.*

Counts as 1 Smart Fiber, 1 Smart Carb, and 1 Smart Protein.

Calories per serving: 232 (with honey); 168 (with Truvia)

## Tropical Delight

*INGREDIENTS*

   1 cup of blueberries (frozen or fresh)

   1 banana

   Handful of fresh spinach

   1 cup of unsweetened coconut milk

   1 tablespoon of honey or 1 to 2 packets of Truvía

*PREPARATION*

Place all ingredients in a blender and blend until smooth.

*Makes 1 serving.*

Counts as 1 Smart Fiber, 1 Smart Carb, and 1 Smart Protein.

Calories per serving: 306 (with honey); 242 (with Truvía)

## A+ Smoothie

### INGREDIENTS

½ cup of canned pumpkin

1 small orange, peeled and cut into small pieces

1 cup of almond milk

1 tablespoon of honey or 1 to 2 packets of Truvía

½ teaspoon of pumpkin pie spice

¼ teaspoon of vanilla extract

### PREPARATION

Place all ingredients in a blender and puree until smooth.

*Makes 1 serving.*

Counts as 1 Smart Fiber, 1 Smart Carb, and 1 Smart Protein.

Calories per serving: 309 (with honey); 245 (with Truvia)

## Yogurt Berry Shake

### INGREDIENTS

½ cup of plain low-fat yogurt

½ cup of unsweetened coconut milk

1 cup of strawberries

½ teaspoon of vanilla extract

1 tablespoon of honey

### PREPARATION

Place all ingredients in a blender and blend until smooth.

*Makes 1 serving.*

Counts as 1 Smart Fiber and 1 Smart Protein.

Calories per serving: 205

## *Peachy Keen Shake*

### INGREDIENTS

    1 cup of almond milk

    $1/3$ cup rolled oats, uncooked

    1 cup of frozen peaches

    1 tablespoon of honey

### PREPARATION

Place all ingredients in a blender and blend until smooth.

*Makes 1 serving.*

Counts as 1 Smart Fiber, 1 Smart Carb, and 1 Smart Protein.

Calories per serving: 286

# BREAKFASTS

For another take on breakfast, I like to make various egg dishes in my skillet—basically egg-white omelets or frittatas. They're never the same thing twice. Sometimes I use tomatoes and peppers, sometimes spinach and mushrooms, but always there's some sort of veggie in the mix. If you like something sweet, try my version of French toast, or even my Fruity Breakfast Salad. There's no guilt to feel, only joy from each bite.

## Veggie Omelet

### INGREDIENTS

Vegetable cooking spray

¼ cup of sliced mushrooms

1 tablespoon of chopped onions

Handful of fresh spinach

4 egg whites, beaten

### PREPARATION

Coat a small skillet with vegetable cooking spray. Place the vegetables in the pan and sauté over medium heat until tender. Set aside. Clean the pan and re-coat with vegetable spray. Pour the beaten egg whites into the pan and cook on medium heat. When the egg whites are cooked through, add the vegetables on top of the eggs and turn half the eggs over the veggies, omelet-style. Heat through for a minute and serve.

*Makes 1 serving.*

Counts as 1 Smart Protein and 1 Smart Fiber.

Calories per serving: 96

## Italian Frittata

### INGREDIENTS

Vegetable cooking spray

¼ cup of chopped tomato

¼ cup of chopped zucchini

1 tablespoon of chopped onion

2 eggs, beaten

½ teaspoon of dried oregano

¼ teaspoon of garlic powder

*PREPARATION*

Coat a small skillet with vegetable cooking spray. Place the vegetables in the pan and sauté over medium heat until tender. Pour the beaten eggs over the veggies in the pan. Sprinkle oregano and garlic powder over the eggs. Cook on medium heat. When the eggs are cooked through, serve.

*Makes 1 serving.*

Counts as 1 Smart Protein and 1 Smart Fiber.

Calories per serving: 174

## Biggest Winner French Toast

*INGREDIENTS*

> 2 tablespoons of almond milk
>
> 2 egg whites
>
> 1 packet of Truvía
>
> ¼ teaspoon of cinnamon
>
> 1 slice of multigrain, gluten-free bread
>
> Vegetable cooking spray

*PREPARATION*

Combine all the ingredients except the bread and cooking spray, and whisk together until well mixed. Soak the bread in the mixture for a few seconds.

Coat a small skillet with vegetable cooking spray. Heat the pan on medium heat. "Fry" the bread in the pan until golden on both sides.

*Makes 1 serving.*

Counts as 1 Smart Carb and 1 Smart Protein.

Calories per serving: 120

## Fruity Breakfast Salad

*INGREDIENTS*

  1 cup of plain nonfat Greek yogurt

  1 cup of unsweetened fresh or frozen strawberries

  1 medium orange, chopped, or 1 kiwifruit, chopped

  1 tablespoon of honey

*PREPARATION*

In a cereal bowl, mix together all the ingredients.

*Makes 1 serving.*

Counts as 1 Smart Protein, 1 Smart Fiber, and 1 Smart Carb.

Calories per serving: 312

# LUNCHES

Carb-loaded, bread-loaded sandwiches for lunch? Get over it. Salads are filling and won't leave you with that 2 p.m. drowsy feeling after lunch. Friends have seen me rummaging through my fridge looking for lettuce so I can make a salad. I don't know what I fear more—running out of toilet paper or running out of salad veggies.

## Chicken Cobb Salad

*INGREDIENTS*

  Lettuce, any type, torn into small pieces, enough to cover a dinner plate or large bowl

  2 green onions, chopped

  1 small tomato, chopped

  1 small carrot, grated

  1 hard-boiled egg, cut into 4 wedges

  1 baked boneless skinless chicken breast, diced into cubes

  2 tablespoons of reduced-calorie or light salad dressing

### PREPARATION

Place the lettuce on the plate and top with the rest of the vegetables, egg, and chicken. Drizzle the salad with the dressing and serve.

*Makes 1 serving.*

Counts as 1 Smart Protein and 1 Smart Fiber.

Calories per serving: 255

## Ranch Lettuce Wraps

### INGREDIENTS

    1 baked boneless skinless chicken breast, diced

    1 green onion, chopped

    1 tablespoon of chopped celery

    1 tablespoon of olive oil

    3 to 4 large lettuce leaves

### PREPARATION

In a small bowl, mix together the chicken, onion, celery, and olive oil. Portion the chicken mixture evenly into the lettuce leaves. Wrap the lettuce around the filling and serve.

*Makes 1 serving.*

Counts as 1 Smart Protein and 1 Smart Fiber.

Calories per serving: 327

## Chicken Almond Salad

### INGREDIENTS

    1 baked boneless skinless chicken breast, diced

    1 tablespoon of slivered almonds

    1 tablespoon of olive oil

2 tablespoons of raspberry vinegar

1 teaspoon of honey

1 medium tomato, quartered slightly so that the tomato is still intact

## PREPARATION

In a small bowl, mix the chicken, almonds, olive oil, raspberry vinegar, and honey. Stuff the chicken mixture into the tomato between the quarters.

*Makes 1 serving.*

Counts as 1 Smart Protein and 1 Smart Fiber.

Calories per serving: 389

## Spinach Salad

### INGREDIENTS

½ bag of baby spinach leaves

½ cucumber, diced

2 tablespoons of chopped onion

½ cup of sliced grape tomatoes

4 slices of fat-free turkey ham, diced

1 tablespoon of olive or flaxseed oil

2 tablespoons of balsamic vinegar

Mrs. Dash to taste

### PREPARATION

Arrange the spinach and vegetables on a plate. Top with the ham. Whisk together the oil, vinegar, and Mrs. Dash to make a salad dressing. Drizzle over the salad.

*Makes 1 serving.*

Counts as 1 Smart Protein and 1 Smart Fiber.

Calories per serving: 309

## Smart Tuna Salad

### INGREDIENTS

    3 to 4 ounces of chunk light tuna

    1 tablespoon of olive oil

    1 teaspoon of Dijon mustard

    1 tablespoon of chopped celery

    1 tablespoon of chopped onion

    1 tablespoon of unsweetened relish

    Lettuce

    4 slices of tomato

### PREPARATION

In a small bowl, mix the tuna with the olive oil, mustard, celery, onion, and relish. Arrange a bed of lettuce on a plate. Spread the tomato slices over the lettuce. Spoon the tuna mixture over the tomato slices.

*Makes 1 serving.*

Counts as 1 Smart Protein and 1 Smart Fiber.

Calories per serving: 302

## Vegetable Bean Salad

### INGREDIENTS

    1 cup of garbanzo beans, drained

    1 cup of red beans or light red kidney beans, drained

    1 red bell pepper, chopped

    ¼ cup of chopped red onion

    Lettuce

*DRESSING INGREDIENTS*

    2 tablespoons of olive oil

    4 tablespoons of red wine vinegar

    1 tablespoon of honey

    ½ teaspoon of Mrs. Dash

    ¼ teaspoon of black pepper

*PREPARATION*

Toss the beans, bell pepper, and onion together in a bowl. In a separate bowl, whisk together the olive oil, vinegar, honey, and spices to make the dressing. Pour the dressing over the beans-veggie mixture and toss. Chill for at least 1 hour, then serve over plates piled generously with lettuce.

*Makes four ½-cup servings (women's portion) or two 1-cup servings (men's portion).*

Counts as 1 Smart Protein and 1 Smart Fiber.

Calories per serving: 213 (for ½-cup serving); 426 (for a 1-cup serving)

## Vegetarian-Style Chili

*INGREDIENTS*

    ½ cup of cooked kidney beans for women; 1 cup for men

    2 tablespoons of salsa

    2 tablespoons of chopped onion

    1 (14.5-ounce) can of stewed tomatoes

    ½ cup of cooked brown rice for women; 1 cup for men

    1 teaspoon of chili powder

    ½ teaspoon of cumin

*PREPARATION*

Put all the ingredients in a saucepan and heat thoroughly over medium heat, about 10 minutes, stirring frequently.

*Makes 1 serving.*

Counts as 1 Smart Protein, 1 Smart Fiber, and 1 Smart Carb.

Calories per serving: 370 (women); 584 (men)

## Taco-Less Salad

*INGREDIENTS*

    1 pound of lean ground turkey

    $2/_3$ cup of water

    1 packet of taco seasoning

    4 cups of chopped lettuce

    2 tablespoons of chopped onion

    Salsa

*PREPARATION*

Brown the ground turkey in a 10" skillet over medium heat; drain. Stir in the water and taco seasoning; heat to boiling. Reduce the heat to low and simmer uncovered for 5 minutes.

    Divide the lettuce and place on four plates. Spoon the turkey mixture over the lettuce. Top with the onions and salsa.

*Makes 4 servings.*

Counts as 1 Smart Protein and 1 Smart Fiber.

Calories per serving: 208

# DINNERS

I'm a chicken breast guy. If I stacked all the boneless, skinless chicken breasts I've eaten since I started working out, I'm sure they'd reach the top of the Empire State Building. For decades, chicken breasts have been the protein currency of dieters everywhere. I know what you're thinking: Chicken breasts are freakin' boring. Yes, they are. I still like to have them for dinner, but I need to acknowledge that other dinner foods do exist.

That's where this section comes in. Join me in varying dinner with everything from lasagna to sweet and sour shrimp to meatloaf. (I've thrown in a chicken breast recipe for old times' sake.)

## Zucchini Lasagna

### INGREDIENTS

    1 pound of lean ground turkey
    3 cloves of garlic, chopped
    1 onion, chopped
    1 (28-ounce) can of crushed tomatoes
    1 teaspoon of dried oregano
    1 teaspoon of dried basil
    $1/8$ teaspoon of pepper
    3 medium zucchini, sliced ¼" thick
    Vegetable cooking spray
    1 cup of fat-free cottage cheese
    ½ cup of fat-free Parmesan cheese
    1 egg

### PREPARATION

In a medium saucepan, brown the turkey over medium heat. Drain to remove any fat. Add the garlic and onion and sauté over medium heat for about 2 minutes. Add the tomatoes, oregano, basil, and pepper. Simmer on low for at least 30 to 40 minutes, uncovered, or until the sauce becomes very thick.

Blot the zucchini slices with a paper towel to remove excess moisture.

Coat a large skillet with vegetable cooking spray. Sauté the zucchini slices on each side until cooked, 1 to 2 minutes per side. Place the slices on paper towels to blot excess moisture.

In a medium bowl, mix together the cheeses and egg. Stir well.

Spread about one-quarter of the sauce on the bottom of a 9x12" casserole dish. Layer one-third of the zucchini slices to cover the sauce. Spread one-third of the cheese mixture over the zucchini. Repeat the layering process twice more. Top with the remaining sauce and cover the lasagna with foil. Bake covered at 375°F for 30 minutes. Let stand 10 minutes before serving.

*Makes 6 servings.*

Counts as 1 Smart Protein and 1 Smart Fiber.

Calories per serving: 283

## *Oriental Chicken with Hot Garlic Sauce*

*INGREDIENTS*

    4 large boneless skinless chicken breasts, cut into chunks

    1 large onion, chopped into large chunks

    2 tablespoons of olive oil

    1 (17-ounce) bag of broccoli florets

*SWEET AND SOUR SAUCE INGREDIENTS*

    10 packets of Truvía

    ½ cup of reduced-sugar ketchup

    ½ cup of distilled white vinegar

    ¼ cup of reduced-sodium soy sauce

    2 teaspoons of garlic powder

    1 to 2 teaspoons of red pepper flakes (depending on your desire for hotness)

*PREPARATION*

Sauté the chicken and onion in the olive oil in a skillet over medium heat until the chicken is cooked throughout and the onion is soft and translucent, about 15 minutes. Add the broccoli. Cook over medium-high heat until the broccoli is heated.

In a small bowl, mix together the sauce ingredients. Pour them into a small skillet and heat over medium heat for 10 minutes, or until the sauce is slightly reduced.

Add the sauce to the chicken mixture. Blend well and heat throughout.

*Makes 4 servings.*

Counts as 1 Smart Protein and 1 Smart Fiber.

Calories per serving: 290

## Stuffed Salmon

*INGREDIENTS*

> 1 cup of cooked brown rice
>
> 1 teaspoon of dried dill
>
> 1 teaspoon of Mrs. Dash
>
> ½ teaspoon of ground pepper
>
> Vegetable cooking spray
>
> 2 salmon fillets with skin on
>
> 1 lemon

*PREPARATION*

In a small bowl, mix together the rice, dill, Mrs. Dash, and pepper. Set aside.

Preheat the oven to 450°F. Coat a cookie sheet with vegetable spray.

Slice the salmon fillets lengthwise, making the cut close to the skin, to create pockets for the rice mixture.

Stuff half the rice mixture into each fillet and place the fillets skin side down on the prepared cookie sheet. Bake the stuffed salmon for 10 minutes per inch thick, or until its flesh is no longer translucent and can easily be broken up with a fork.

Remove the fish from the oven, squeeze lemon juice over each piece, and serve.

*Makes 2 servings.*

Counts as 1 Smart Protein and 1 Smart Carb.

Calories per serving: 184

## Easy Roast Turkey

*INGREDIENTS*

> 1 turkey breast
>
> Poultry seasoning
>
> Mrs. Dash
>
> Vegetable cooking spray

### PREPARATION

Preheat the oven to 350°F.

Sprinkle the turkey breast with poultry seasoning and Mrs. Dash. Spray the breast lightly with vegetable cooking spray. Bake in a glass baking dish uncovered for about 40 minutes or until the turkey is cooked through and the juices run clear.

*Makes 2 servings.*

Counts as 1 Smart Protein.

Calories per serving: 207

## Lean and Tasty Meatloaf

### INGREDIENTS

Vegetable cooking spray

1½ pounds of lean ground turkey

1 cup of almond milk

1 tablespoon of Worcestershire sauce

1 small onion, chopped

½ teaspoon of dried sage leaves

½ teaspoon of Mrs. Dash

½ teaspoon of ground mustard

¼ teaspoon of pepper

¼ teaspoon of garlic powder

1 egg, beaten lightly

1 cup of uncooked oatmeal

### PREPARATION

Preheat the oven to 375°F. Coat a 9x5" loaf pan with vegetable cooking spray.

Combine the rest of the ingredients in a large mixing bowl and mix well. Spoon the mixture into the prepared loaf pan and shape into a loaf. Bake uncovered for 1 hour 15 minutes to 1 hour 30 minutes.

*Makes 6 servings.*

Counts as 1 Smart Protein and 1 Smart Carb.

Calories per serving: 252

## Sweet and Sour Shrimp

### INGREDIENTS

Vegetable cooking spray

1 pound of fresh shrimp, peeled, cleaned

½ cup of sliced green bell pepper

½ cup of sliced red bell pepper

¼ cup of lite soy sauce

1 teaspoon of minced garlic

½ cup of sugar-free pineapple syrup or sugar-free maple syrup

1 tablespoon of white vinegar

1 tablespoon of Truvía

¼ teaspoon of powdered ginger

### PREPARATION

Coat a large skillet with vegetable cooking spray. Add the shrimp and sauté over medium heat until they are bright pink and opaque. Add the green and red bell pepper, soy sauce, and garlic and sauté for 1 to 2 minutes.

In a small saucepan, combine the pineapple syrup, vinegar, Truvía, and ginger. Stir well to combine and bring to a full boil. Pour the sauce over the shrimp and vegetable mixture in the skillet. Heat thoroughly and serve.

*Makes 4 servings.*

Counts as 1 Smart Protein and 1 Smart Fiber.

Calories per serving: 198

# SIDE DISHES

I have a mantra that says "It's not a meal without a side dish." I should add "a healthy side dish," since the sides you commonly find are French fries, high-fat potato salad, mashed potatoes, and other poor choices. Wash it all down with a soda, and you've just drowned in a sea of fattening carbs. I've got some side dishes here that you'll love, and you won't miss the junk.

## Quinoa Apple Salad

### INGREDIENTS

2 cups of water

1 cup of quinoa, rinsed and drained

1 cup of peeled, chopped apples

¼ cup of sliced almonds, toasted

1 tablespoon of olive oil

2 tablespoons of raspberry vinegar

1 teaspoon of Truvia

### PREPARATION

In a medium saucepan, bring the water to a boil and add the quinoa. Cook for 10 to 15 minutes over medium-low heat, until the water is absorbed and the quinoa is tender. Let the quinoa cool, then combine it with the apples and almonds.

Combine the olive oil, vinegar, and Truvía in a small bowl. Toss it with the quinoa mixture and chill for at least 30 minutes before serving.

*Makes 4 servings.*

Counts as 1 Smart Carb and 1 Smart Fiber.

Calories per serving: 238

## "Fried" Rice

INGREDIENTS

 2 cups of cooked brown rice

 2 tablespoons of lite soy sauce

 1 large scallion, chopped

 ½ red bell pepper, chopped

 ½ zucchini, chopped

 ½ large portobello mushroom, chopped

PREPARATION

Add the rice to a large frying pan set over medium heat and start heating. Add the soy sauce. If the rice seems dry, add a tablespoon or two of water. Add the vegetables to the rice. The mushroom will give off a tasty liquid as it cooks.

Heat the mixture through until the vegetables are tender. Remove from the heat and serve.

*Makes 4 servings.*

Counts as 1 Smart Carb and 1 Smart Fiber.

Calories per serving: 127 (for ½-cup serving for women); 255 (for 1-cup serving for men)

## Spinach Chips

INGREDIENTS

 1 bag of spinach

 Vegetable cooking spray

 Mrs. Dash

PREPARATION

Preheat the oven to 300°F. Line a large sheet pan with parchment paper.

Wash and thoroughly dry the spinach. Tear the larger leaves into 1" to 2" strips.

Place the spinach leaves in a single layer on the parchment paper. Spritz lightly with vegetable cooking spray and sprinkle with Mrs. Dash.

Bake until the spinach is dry and has darkened slightly, 15 to 20 minutes. Remove immediately from the pan and transfer to a serving dish. Serve immediately, or store in a brown paper bag at room temperature for up to 3 days.

*Makes 1 serving.*

Counts as 1 Smart Fiber.

Calories per serving: 75

## Maple Orange Mashed Sweet Potatoes

*INGREDIENTS*

2 medium-sized sweet potatoes, peeled, roughly chopped

¼ cup of almond milk

1 teaspoon of pumpkin pie spice

1 tablespoon of honey

¼ cup of sugar-free orange marmalade

2 tablespoons of sugar-free maple syrup

*PREPARATION*

Fill a large pot with water and bring it to a boil. Add the sweet potatoes and boil until tender, about 15 minutes. Drain and return to the pan.

Add the milk, pumpkin pie spice, honey, orange marmalade, and maple syrup. Mash until smooth. Heat thoroughly and serve.

*Makes 2 servings.*

Counts as 1 Smart Carb.

Calories per serving: 172

## Sweet Potato Fries

*INGREDIENTS*

4 large sweet potatoes, cut into wedges

Vegetable cooking spray

2 to 3 tablespoons of sesame seeds

1 teaspoon of Mrs. Dash

*PREPARATION*

Preheat the oven to 400°F. Coat a baking sheet with vegetable cooking spray.

Spray the potato wedges with vegetable cooking spray. Place them in a large bowl and toss them with the sesame seeds and Mrs. Dash.

Place the potatoes on the prepared baking sheet and bake for about 30 minutes, or until fork-tender.

*Makes 4 servings.*

Counts as 1 Smart Carb.

Calories per serving: 131

## Dolvett's Mock Mashed Potatoes

*INGREDIENTS*

1½ cups of fat-free, sodium-free chicken broth

1 head of cauliflower, cut into bite-size pieces, thick stems removed

4 parsnips, peeled and chopped

1 small onion, finely chopped

2 medium garlic cloves, smashed

2 teaspoons Mrs. Dash, plus more as needed

White pepper, to taste

*PREPARATION*

Heat the chicken broth in a large saucepan with a tight-fitting lid over medium-high heat until simmering. Add the cauliflower, parsnips, onion, garlic, Mrs. Dash, and pepper to taste.

Bring to a boil. Reduce the heat to low. Cover and simmer until the vegetables are tender, about 20 minutes.

Transfer the mixture, including the liquid, to a blender or food processor. Process until smooth. Taste and season with additional Mrs. Dash and pepper as needed, then transfer to a serving bowl.

*Makes 4 servings.*

Counts as 1 Smart Fiber and 1 Smart Carb.

Calories per serving: 163

## Veggistrone

*INGREDIENTS*

> 4 cups of fat-free, sodium-free chicken broth
>
> 1 cup of water
>
> 1 (15-ounce) can of tomato sauce
>
> 1 (14-ounce) can of diced tomatoes
>
> 1 bay leaf
>
> 1 cup of chopped onion
>
> 1 cup of chopped celery
>
> 1 cup of chopped carrots
>
> 2 cloves of garlic, minced
>
> 2 cups of chopped cabbage
>
> 1 cup of chopped cauliflower
>
> 2 cups of frozen green beans
>
> 2 cups of chopped fresh kale
>
> 6 tablespoons of fat-free Parmesan cheese

*PREPARATION*

Add the broth, water, tomato sauce, tomatoes, and bay leaf to a large soup pan and cook over medium heat. Add the onion, celery, carrots, and garlic, and cook, stirring frequently, until the veggies are tender, about 15 minutes. Add the cabbage, cauliflower, and green beans, and cook, stirring occasionally, about 10 minutes more. Simmer for another 20 to 25 minutes. Stir in the kale and simmer for 10 minutes more.

Discard the bay leaf. Spoon the soup into bowls and top each portion with 1 tablespoon of Parmesan cheese.

The soup will keep in the fridge for 4 to 5 days or in the freezer for 6 months.

*Makes 6 servings.*

Counts as 1 Smart Fiber.

Calories per serving: 114

## Fruit Treat

*INGREDIENTS*

1 cup of mixed fresh berries

1 tablespoon of nonfat plain yogurt

2 teaspoons of honey

*PREPARATION*

Put the berries in a cereal bowl. Mix together the yogurt and honey and drizzle over the top of the fruit.

*Makes 1 serving.*

Counts as 1 Smart Fiber.

Calories per serving: 120

# MODIFY YOUR FAVORITE RECIPES

Some people work their whole lives at improving their golf swings, but my new skill is much more practical. I'm talking about modifying your favorite recipes from fatty versions to diet-friendly versions that are lower in fat, sugar, and calories but still taste fantastic. Granted, if you're stuck on mega cinnamon rolls, for example, you're probably not going to come up with a healthy mega cinnamon roll. But if you can adjust your attitude a bit and be willing to make a few modifications, you will be surprised at how delicious and satisfying your recipes will be—worthy of using them as your cheat meals. Here are some tips:

If you're incorporating baked goods into your cheat meals, why not cut the sugar and fat? It's easy. Substitute applesauce, ripe bananas, or pureed peaches for the oil or butter and sugar in muffins, quick breads, cakes, and other baked goods. (When you decrease or replace some of the fats in the recipe, lower the oven temperature for baking by about 25 degrees. Baking at a lower temperature helps keep baked goods moist. After baking and cooling, refrigerate the items to maintain freshness.)

Try using light butter or margarine in lieu of the full-fat version. For example, if the recipe asks you to cream butter, use trans-fat-free tub margarine in place of stick margarine or butter to lower saturated fat.

Cut the calories, as well as the fat and cholesterol, in recipes by using egg whites for whole eggs. In baking, substitute two egg whites for the first whole egg and one egg white for each additional egg. Using egg whites can save you around 50 calories for each egg substituted.

Want to whip up something chocolaty on your cheat days? Forget regular baking chocolate; it adds 145 calories and 15 grams of fat per one 1-ounce square. Instead, use 3 tablespoons of unsweetened cocoa powder mixed with 2 teaspoons of water. This substitution adds only 45 calories and 5 grams of fat, and replaces the fattening ounce of baking chocolate. Plus, this lower-calorie, lower-fat sub works deliciously for cakes, brownies, and puddings.

Enhance flavor with sweet spices such as cinnamon, nutmeg, or cloves, and with extracts such as vanilla, almond, and coconut. None has any calories.

Finally, use nonfat Greek yogurt as a substitute for fats, in addition to enjoying it as a healthy Smart Protein. For example, ¾ cup of Greek yogurt can stand in for 1 cup of oil; 1 cup of Greek yogurt can substitute for 1 cup of sour cream or mayonnaise. One of my favorite things to do with Greek yogurt is to turn it into "ice cream." Try the following recipe for a tasty dessert or snack.

## Dolvett's Creamy Frozen Yogurt

*INGREDIENTS*

2 cups of sliced fresh strawberries

$1/3$ cup of sugar-free or low-sugar strawberry preserves

½ cup of granulated Truvía

2 cups of fat-free plain Greek yogurt

1 teaspoon of vanilla extract

*PREPARATION*

Before you get started, read and follow the instructions for the ice cream maker you have. Some of the newer models require that the freezer container be frozen prior to making the ice cream.

Put the strawberries in a blender and blend until they are pureed. Add the sugar-free strawberry preserves and Truvía and blend for about 30 seconds. Then add the yogurt and vanilla extract and blend until the mixture is smooth. (You can also use a food processor.)

Place the mixture into the ice cream container with the blades in place. Put the lid on and run the motor. Let the yogurt mixture freeze to ice cream consistency. It should take about 30 minutes.

You can eat the frozen yogurt after preparing it, or freeze it. If you freeze it, the frozen yogurt gets hard. Let it soften at room temperature for about 10 minutes prior to eating.

*Makes 2 servings.*

Counts as 1 Smart Protein and 1 Smart Fiber. You can also enjoy a cup of this frozen yogurt as one of your snacks.

Calories per serving: 222 calories

Okay—have fun with these mouth-watering recipes and my supereasy 21-day plan. They will help you get rid of fat, hunger, and cravings, plus help you feel great!

Now, if your goal is to get a tighter, more defined, superfit body, then it's time to talk about my workout. It's designed to make further metabolic changes in your body—with some calorie-blasting, super-fat-burning moves that can be done in as little as 48 minutes a session.

# Part Two

## *Change Your Body, One Rep at a Time*

# 6 My Make-It-Burn Exercises

As a personal trainer, I've always taken pride in training people in different ways. One day, a very close friend of mine suggested that, rather than train my clients with different styles, I create a single, foolproof training method that would work for everyone, something that I could put my personal stamp on. His suggestion made sense but would prove to be a real challenge. After all, the health and fitness industry is always evolving—new inventions, new gadgets, and new training systems, the latest and the greatest this, that, or the other. But since I love a challenge, I applied what I knew to make it happen.

The result, called Pure Energy, was a high-intensity circuit-training system, led by trainers and performed in a class with a live DJ spinning fun, high-powered dance music. The concept behind the system was "cardio meets strength training." People did intervals of intense cardio work punctuated by intervals of strength training and resistance exercises. All fitness levels could participate.

The meshing of cardio with strength was definitely important. A lot of guys go to the gym to lift weights, but they don't do any cardio. Result: They aren't really lean; they're bulky. A lot of women just go to the gym and say, "Okay, I don't want muscle; I'd rather do cardio." Ladies, please: Don't be afraid of lifting weights. Nothing feels better than a nice toned body, so you've got to add weights to your routine. They give you a sexy, lean body. In all honesty, everybody needs both strength training and cardio. My approach mixes and matches both.

The response to Pure Energy blew me away. People were dropping weight, trimming inches, and getting superdefined by following this system several times a week. The classes were so popular that the workout was voted Best Workout in the Southeast. Of course, I was pumped, and I knew I was on to something, so this became my signature workout, and I use it to this day. The workout you'll do as part of following the 3-1-2-1 Diet is the same workout as Pure Energy, only condensed into just 48 minutes.

The brevity of this workout is a plus. Time is cited again and again as the number one reason why so many Americans do not exercise regularly or at all. In today's crazy-busy world, it's easy to neglect yourself, and exercise is often the first thing to fall through the cracks of our hectic lives.

That's all fine, but I don't care how hectic your lifestyle is. You can always squeeze in 48 minutes of exercise a day. Going back and forth from your couch to the fridge several times a day and calling this "doing laps" doesn't cut it. Don't hang out with me if you decide to try that one out!

My routine is not only time efficient; it's also very productive. In other words, you do more in less time and still get exceptional body-shaping, body-toning results in the end. This workout gives you a unique sequence of exercises designed to reshape your most troublesome body parts and burn fat in the very same workout.

And 1 day a week, I'll ask you to do something for "active fun"—something completely out of the normal: Go hiking, ride a bicycle, play volleyball, swim, or whatever it takes to engage your muscles in a whole new way.

Speaking of fun, exercise should be something you enjoy doing. Right now, you're probably shaking your head and thinking that exercise and having fun at the same time doesn't make sense, that it's impossible. But take it from me: It's all in how you approach it. You've got to take the *work* out of working out. How? By really falling in love with this thing called exercise. Have an attitude adjustment to turn working out into a natural part of your life. Don't let being active be a burden. Instead think of it more like "that fun thing I do." You can do this workout to your favorite music, too, and that makes it powerfully fun.

I love music, and I love to sing, always have. So whenever I set out to exercise, I always have my iPod with a playlist of my favorite tunes. Those tunes inspire me to either kick up my intensity or hold steady and groove on my surroundings. So basically, music inspires me to move my body to its optimal potential and enjoy the ride.

Music truly does make a difference in the quality of your workouts. Studies show that people exercise harder with music, especially when that music is fast-paced and up-tempo. Of course, the harder you exercise, the more fat you burn. People also report that the exercise is more enjoyable when done to music.

Along with having fun, you'll get fast results. After even a week or two of exercising like this, you'll notice that you're leaner and shapelier than ever. The workout is designed to address all three "fat patterns" commonly seen on the human form: the *abdomen pattern*, in which fat collects mostly around the waist; the *hip/thigh pattern*, in which fat collects around the buttocks and thighs; and the *uniform pattern*, in which fat appears to be distributed uniformly on the body. This workout combines special body-sculpting exercises with cardio moves to reshape your entire body.

This workout is convenient too. Studies show that one of the main reasons people drop out of exercise programs is inconvenience. Well, you can do this workout right in the comfort of your own home—or if you wish, at a gym. I'll give you exercise options you can do at just about any gym.

## AFFIRM TO GET FIRM: IT HURTS TO LOOK GOOD...

I'm in pain every day—but not "bad" pain. I'm talking about the muscle pain you get after an intense workout. That pain is a positive signal. It tells you that your body is in a state of transformation because you worked it well. It's also the pain you feel in those last few reps of an exercise when you pushed yourself a little farther. Start welcoming muscle soreness and equating pain as signposts to a brand-new super-fit body. Every time you feel muscle soreness, visualize the new shape you'll soon be in.

## I Did It on Dolvett's Program!

I'm sixty years old, and I heard that it was tough to lose weight as you age, so I was a little reluctant to try to lose the 25 pounds I needed to lose. I started with Dolvett's workout 4 times a week. Then I increased it to 6 times a week. The workout fit right into my schedule, and I liked the idea that I could do cardio and strength training all in one exercise session. At the same time, I learned that building muscle would boost my metabolism, despite my age. So I started the 3-1-2-1 Diet.

Within 6 weeks, I had a buff body and flatter, defined abs. I realized another benefit of the workout: I could still lose weight even with the 2 cheat days. I think I was losing more fat because I was gaining metabolism-boosting muscle.

Once I started the diet, I noticed, too, that I had more energy for workouts and day-to-day activities. Even after my workouts, I felt invigorated and energized. I kept at it all—diet and workout—because I was so fired up. I lost the 25 pounds and feel like I'm in my twenties. I'm continually amazed by what my sixty-year-old body can do!

My tips:

- Map out your meals for the week. I'm pretty analytical, so on Sunday, I write out what I'm going to eat for the week. This makes grocery shopping easy and helps me plan my cheats. There's no room for error when you plan your meals.
- Switch up your exercise routine. Every 2 weeks, I add something new to my workouts. For example, I might try a new class at the gym or go for a hike when the weather is nice.
- Keep building muscle. Don't be afraid of lifting weights. It maintains muscle mass, which in turn burns more calories and keeps your weight off.

*—Martin S.*

# GEAR UP TO GET GOING

If you do this workout at home, there are few inexpensive items you'll need to gather together.

## Exercise Mat

For floor exercises, you'll need a dense foam mat to cushion your body during the workout. The mat you choose should be comfortable, yet provide support for your spine, so look for one that is firm enough to hold your body weight without collapsing under it.

## Flat Exercise Bench

Although not a necessity, having a weight bench will give you more exercise options and makes certain exercises easier to complete. When shopping for a bench, look for stability above comfort. Unless you plan on fastening it to the floor, steer clear of lightweight benches that may tip over. Other features include adjustable barbell racks and the ability to incline and decline. If you don't get a bench, a chair or ottoman works great for home use.

## Set of Dumbbells (ranging from 10 to 30 pounds)

I began weight training when I was fourteen years old, and the first piece of equipment I ever picked up was the dumbbell. Since then, I have worked out on practically every type of equipment. I've experimented with every method of training, and I've followed many exercise philosophies. Through it all, I always gravitate back to dumbbells, which have been around since the time of the ancient Greeks. You won't see these old-fashioned training tools on infomercials; they just aren't fancy enough. But there isn't a better, or easier, piece of equipment for getting results.

You can do just about any strength-training move with the trusty old dumbbell. It can be used in a varying range of motion, it can sculpt any body part, and it promotes overall body fitness. The right combination of dumbbell exercises can enhance muscular strength, give you more muscular endurance, and change your body composition so that you have less fat and more lean muscle in all the right places. Think of the dumbbell as an all-purpose fitness tool.

## Adjustable Barbell

Another chunk of iron you can lift, instead of boxes of cookies and gallons of ice cream, is the barbell. Like dumbbells, barbells are free weights with which you can work just about any part of your body. Besides giving you more options for exercise, barbells last forever with little maintenance, don't take up much floor space, and are inexpensive. You'll want to gradually increase the weight you use, so purchase an adjustable barbell that comes with several sizes of plates. Men generally prefer barbells; women seem to prefer dumbbells. If you don't want to add a barbell to your home gym, that's okay, since any barbell exercise can usually be done with dumbbells.

## Resistance Bands

I am a big fan of resistance bands. These tools are inexpensive and versatile. They can be used anywhere and easily packed into a suitcase if you're traveling out of town. They're made of stretchy rubber, and many are produced in latex or latex-free versions. Resistance bands normally come with easy-to-grip handles.

With resistance bands, you've got to be familiar with how to get the most body-sculpting resistance. The available levels of resistance are usually light, medium, or heavy, and the bands are coded by color (for most brands, green is light; red is heavy). Bands provide "variable resistance." This means, for example, that they might equal 15 pounds of resistance when stretched out but only 5 pounds with no tension. You don't get much benefit without tension on the band. The tighter the band, the harder and more intense the exercise. A set of bands of different levels of resistance lets you perform virtually the same routine you might do at a gym using weights or machines.

In my routine, you'll find some exercises in which you have the option to use dumbbells or a resistance band. For some workouts, you may feel like using the band; for others, your dumbbells. Feel free to use either or switch it up from workout to workout. I like giving folks options and choices.

## Stopwatch

My workout moves quickly, involving cardio and the exercises described below. It puts you through a series of timed cardio and strength-training circuits, so you'll need to have a stopwatch or a clock with a second hand—any sort of timepiece you can see easily while working out.

# CARDIO OPTIONS AT HOME

You'll be mixing in fat-burning cardio with your strength-training moves, so you have a couple of options here if you're working out at home:

Standard floor exercises such as running in place or doing jumping jacks can provide a good cardio workout using no equipment. Or you can jump rope, if you want something really vigorous. It's an intense cardio workout. Have stairs in your home? If so, climbing up and down your staircase will do the trick. Weather permitting, you can even do this workout outdoors. For cardio, run in the park or around the block. If you're near a beach, run on the sand. I use sand frequently in workouts. Sand adds a resistance that forces you to work twice as hard to run. If you're working twice as hard, you're burning more in a shorter period of time!

If you want some cardio equipment for your home gym, there are lots of options, though they can be a little pricey. Here's a rundown (all of these are available at gyms too):

## Treadmill

Walking or jogging on a treadmill is a terrific cardio workout. Select a model that has an incline; this is good for sculpting your thighs and back. And once you exceed a speed of 3.5 miles per hour, raise that incline or start jogging to boost your intensity and fat burn. A 3 percent incline provides the calorie burn of running outdoors.

## Elliptical Trainer

An elliptical trainer is a combination treadmill and stepping machine. Your feet and legs move in a semicircle-type pattern, rather than straight up and down, and this helps relieve pressure from your joints. By the way, I'm pretty sure this device was invented by a hamster to get back at the human race.

## Stationary Bike

These machines are lighter and less expensive than treadmills and are great not only for cardio but also for working the thighs. Buy a bike that has mechanisms that let you easily control the resistance. Make sure you know how to properly adjust the bike. How can you tell if a stationary bike is right for you—and feels right? Take it for a "test ride." Try it out. Different manufacturers make bikes with different seat heights, and not all seats can be adjusted, so make sure you can fit comfortably on the bike and that it feels smooth while exercising.

## Stair Climber (Stepper)

Fairly cheap and compact, stair climbers have more hard-core fans than any other machine, and I'm one of them. Steppers provide a great lower-body workout, along with cardio benefits. If you want to get a stair climber, get a good one. Cheap climbers tend to clatter and often have flimsy handrails, and the resistance between steps sometimes doesn't feel right.

## Rowing Machine

Rowing is supereasy, something anyone can do. It's a low-impact way to get in shape because you're sitting down and using your upper-body strength. At the same time, rowing is perfect for cardio fitness and endurance. Depending on how hard you row, you can burn anywhere between 400 and 1,000 calories per hour. That high caloric burn makes rowing very effective for weight loss. To get the most from rowing, keep your back straight as you pull back and reach forward, and make sure to keep your abs contracted.

# MY BODY-SCULPTING MOVES

On the pages that follow, I'll show you how to do all my best body-sculpting moves. Each move is part of the routine you'll read about in the next chapter. For now, I'd like you to read through this section and get familiar with each of the exercises. Practice them, too, so that they become second nature. In the next chapter you'll put the moves together in my specifically formulated 48-minute routine that will tone your body, burn fat, and get you back into those jeans you wore in high school!

## Lower-Body Exercises

### *SQUATS*

*Squats are the most effective exercise you can do to tone your legs and booty. There are lots of ways you can perform squats, from simply using your own body weight to adding resistance such as dumbbells or barbells. If you are a gym member, your facility probably has several different types of squat machines.*

To begin, grasp either a weighted bar or two dumbbells. If using a bar, drape it across your shoulders behind your neck. If using dumbbells, hold them at your sides, palms facing inward.

Stand with your legs just slightly apart, so they are at least even with your shoulders. Point your toes forward. Stand straight to maintain good posture. Breathe naturally throughout the exercise. Tighten your abdominal muscles.

Bend your body forward slightly, and lower your body as if you are going to sit on a chair without sitting completely down. Lower until your thighs are parallel to the floor.

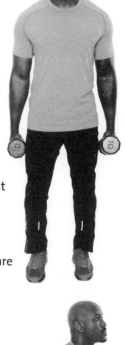

Hold that position for a few seconds, push off from your heels, and return to the upright position.

Continue this motion for the number of minutes designated in the routine. Over time, increase the number of repetitions, or weights for maximum results, as well as the time.

## RESISTANCE BAND SQUATS

Wrap the band around a secure point, such as a pole or stair railing.

Face the pole. Stand with your legs slightly wider than shoulder width. Point your toes forward. Stand straight to maintain good posture. Breathe naturally throughout the exercise. Tighten your abdominal muscles.

Grasp the resistance band's handles and pull the band toward you.

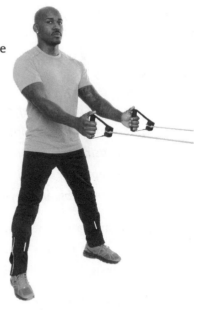

Bend your knees and lower your body so that your knees are parallel to the floor. Hold that position for a few seconds, push off from your heels, and return to the upright position.

Continue the exercise for the number of minutes designated in the routine. Over time, increase the tension on the band for maximum results.

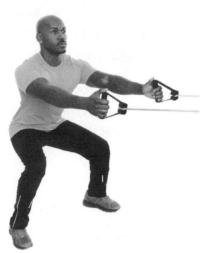

## FORWARD LUNGE

*Lunges work all the major muscles of the legs and hips at the same time, they lengthen and tone those muscles, and they burn a ton of calories. Not only do they strengthen your glutes and quadriceps, but they also strengthen your knee joints and help with stabilization and balance. They can be done with no equipment. Lunges require a great deal of energy, which raises your heart rate. They are a multijoint movement, which means they use joints other than the knees. Whether you want to tone your lower body or strengthen your joints, lunges are the perfect exercise.*

To begin, stand with your feet at approximately shoulder width apart, with your toes pointed forward. Take dumbbells of equal weight in your hands and allow your arms to hang straight down at your sides as you perform the exercise.

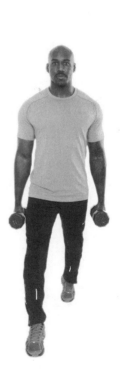

Step forward on your right foot. Bend your right knee while keeping your knee pointed in the same direction as your foot.

Keep your torso upright as you continue to bend your right knee until your right thigh is parallel to the floor and your left knee is nearly touching the floor. Make sure that your right knee does not extend beyond your toes.

Pause briefly in this position and then return to your starting position. Repeat the exercise on your left leg. Continue lunging, alternating legs, for the number of minutes designated in the routine.

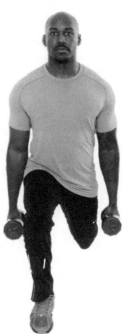

## *BACKWARD LUNGE*

To begin, stand with your feet fairly close together with your toes pointed forward. Take dumbbells of equal weight in your hands and allow your arms to hang straight down at your sides as you perform the exercise.

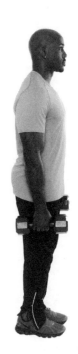

Step back with your left leg onto your left toe. Bend your left knee while keeping your knee pointed in the same direction as your foot.

Keep your torso upright as you continue to bend your right knee until your right thigh is parallel to the floor and your left knee is nearly touching the floor behind you.

Pause briefly in this position and then return to your starting position. Repeat the exercise on your left leg. Continue, alternating legs, for the number of minutes designated in the routine.

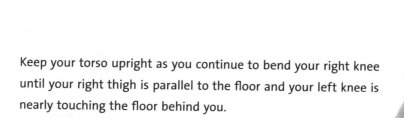

## RESISTANCE BAND LUNGES

Wrap the band around a secure point, such as a pole or stair railing.

Face the pole. Stand with your feet fairly close together. Point your toes forward. Stand straight to maintain good posture. Breathe naturally throughout the exercise. Tighten your abdominal muscles.

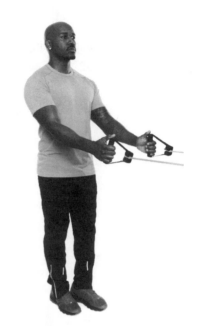

Grasp the resistance band's handles, and pull the band toward you. Step forward with your left foot until your left thigh is almost parallel to the floor. Return to the starting position and perform the exercise on your right leg.

Continue, alternating legs, for the amount of time designated in the routine.

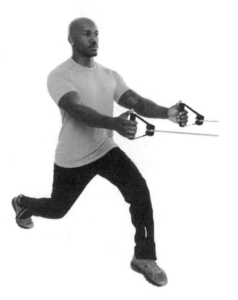

## DEAD LIFTS

*The dead lift is a great all-over exercise. It can really develop firm, beautiful muscles by working the back, thighs, butt, arms, and forearms, as well as the abs. Few other exercises do as much as the dead lift.*

To begin, use either a weighted barbell or two dumbbells of equal weight. If using a barbell, take an overhand grip and hold it across your upper thighs. If using dumbbells, take an overhand grip and hold them as shown in the photograph. Place your feet approximately shoulder-width apart, with your toes pointed slightly outward.

Keeping your legs straight, bend your body at the hips. Keep your head down and look at the floor. Lower the weights to the floor.

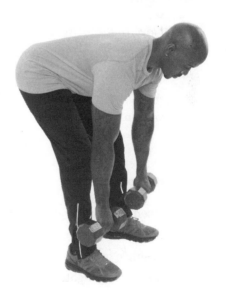

Next, pushing with your heels, begin to return to the starting position. As you do this, begin to push your hips forward. When you reach the top of the lift, squeeze your butt and pull the weight into your body, while keeping your back straight.

Continue performing the dead lift with proper form for the number of minutes designated in the routine.

## SUMO SQUATS

*I love this exercise because it tones those often-flabby inner thighs and glutes so well. In addition, the move can be performed anywhere, and you can do it with or without a dumbbell. Don't let the name throw you; you won't turn into a sumo wrestler, just a sexier, more defined version of yourself.*

Hold one dumbbell with both hands at your pelvis.

Stand with your legs wide apart, wider than your shoulders. Point your toes outward. Stand straight to maintain good posture. Breathe naturally throughout the exercise. Tighten your abdominal muscles.

Bend your knees and lower your torso toward the floor until your thighs are parallel to the floor.

Hold that position for a few seconds, and return to the upright position.

Continue performing the sumo squat with proper form for the amount of time designated in the routine. Over time, increase the number of repetitions, or weights, or time for maximum results.

## HAMSTRING LIFTS WITH RESISTANCE BANDS

*This exercise targets the hamstrings at the back of the upper legs. Unfortunately, the hamstrings are not sexy muscles, so a lot of people neglect them. However, get your hamstrings in shape and your body will respond. Running, walking, reaching, jumping, and other functional moves will become easier. Plus, your legs will look sleeker in shorts when you have well-developed hamstrings.*

Place your toes through the handles of the resistance band. Then lie on your back on an exercise mat or other soft surface and place your hands at your sides. Have someone stand on the middle of the band to secure it to the floor. Bend your knees.

Keeping your hips on the floor, straighten your legs, bringing your feet back toward your head, getting a good stretch in your hamstrings. Return to the starting position and continue the exercise for the amount of time designated in the routine.

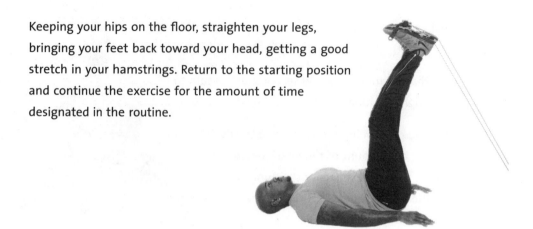

## Upper-Body Large-Muscle Workout

### PUSH-UPS

*What I love about push-ups is that they employ your body weight as resistance, so you don't have to use exercise equipment, and you can do them anywhere, any time. They're a terrific way to tone and sculpt your upper body, particularly your chest and triceps, if done properly.*

Lie facedown on an exercise mat or other soft surface. Extend your legs out behind you while bracing yourself with your hands. If you wish to do a modified push-up, kneel on the mat, making sure your back is straight. Position your hands on the floor slightly more than shoulder width apart and keep your abdominal muscles tight.

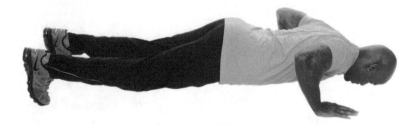

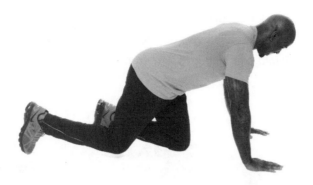

Lower yourself to the point just before your body touches the floor. Then extend your arms to push yourself up from the floor. Push up and down like this for the designated amount of time in the routine.

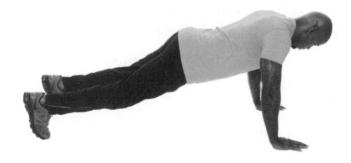

## PLANK

*You don't need a lot of equipment to get in a good workout around your core. When I say "core," I'm referring to your torso, your abs, and all the way around your back muscles and lower back. A lot of people care about the "show muscles," like the chest or the thighs. But the core is the brain of the body. If you have a strong core, you'll be able to improve the rest of your fitness. That means you can lift more, run faster, and run longer. I feel the very best exercise for toning and strengthening the core is the plank. It's my go-to exercise for a strong center.*

Lie facedown on an exercise mat or other soft surface. Hold your upper-body weight on your forearms and elbows on the mat, and align your shoulders directly over your elbows. Hold your hands in fists front of you.

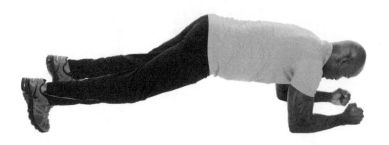

Stretch your legs straight out behind you and rest on your toes, as if you are going to do a push-up. Now push your butt up in the air until your body is in a bit of an arc and your buttocks are pointing up toward the ceiling.

Hold this position for 30 seconds. Tightening your abdominal muscles will help you stay in the plank position.

## ALTERNATING PUSH-UPS AND PLANKS

For a wickedly intense workout, do both exercises in an alternating fashion, without resting between them, for the designated amount of time in the routine.

## CHEST BUTTERFLY PRESS

*There are three effective ways you can tone and build up your chest: with a chest-press exercise machine, with dumbbells, or with resistance bands. Here, I demonstrate how to perform this exercise with dumbbells and resistance bands. The exercise works all the pectoral muscles (chest), which help with posture and strength. Other muscles affected are the triceps (back of upper arms) and deltoids (rear shoulders).*

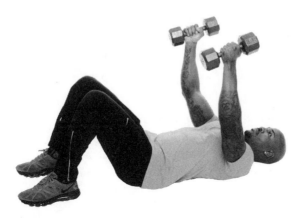

Lie on your back on an exercise mat or other soft surface. Bend your knees. Grasp dumbbells of equal weight in your hands. Bring your weights up so your arms are straight and the palms of your hands face each other.

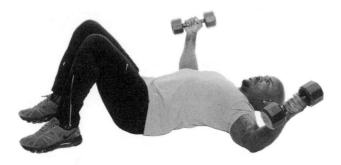

Bring your arms out to your sides in an arc. Get a good stretch in your chest. Slowly bring your arms back to the start position and repeat the exercise.

## CHEST BUTTERFLY PRESS WITH A RESISTANCE BAND

Wrap a resistance band around a pole, tree, bedpost, or other sturdy stationary object, so that it is lined up with the middle of your chest muscles. Take a split stance, as shown, and grasp the handles of the resistance band in both hands. Step forward to get some tension in the band. Begin with your arms extended out to your sides.

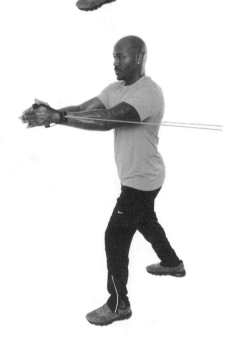

Slowly bring your arms together out in front of you. Contract your chest muscles in this position. Then return to the start position and repeat.

## DUMBBELL CHEST PRESS

*Chest presses involving dumbbells or resistance bands zero in on your chest muscles to shock them into growth. Both are excellent variations, due in part to their full resistance throughout the exercise and their allowance of a full range of motion.*

Lie on your back on an exercise mat or other soft surface. Grasp dumbbells of equal weight in your hands and hold at your sides, elbows bent.

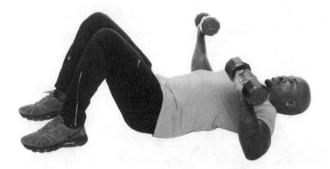

Press the dumbbells up over your head, arms extended.

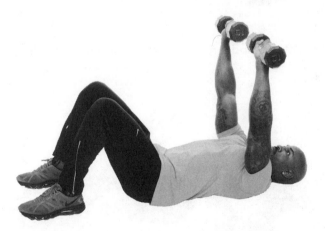

Slowly lower the dumbbells to the start position. Repeat this motion for the designated amount of time in the routine.

## DUMBBELL PULLOVERS

*A pullover is an exercise that builds muscle strength and definition in the back and chest. You can perform the movement with a dumbbell or resistance bands. Both are easy to do but require strict attention to form for best results.*

Lie on your back on an exercise mat or other soft surface, while holding a dumbbell with both hands behind your head with a slight bend in your arms.

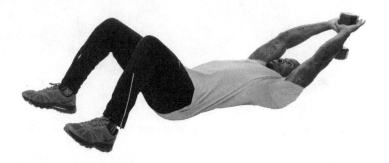

Maintain the bent-arm position, and bring the weight forward in an arc toward your knees.

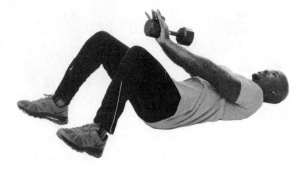

Slowly bring the dumbbell back to the starting position.

Repeat the movement for the designated amount of time in the routine.

## DUMBBELL ROWS

*Rowing exercises are very popular body-sculpting moves. In my workout, you use dumbbells and resistance bands to isolate your back muscles and stress the latissimus dorsi (the "lats"). Both exercises will shape your back and help you give you a V taper, which is, simply put, a wider chest and small waist. It's a shapely, sexy look that's easy to accomplish by being faithful to diet and exercise.*

Grasp a dumbbell in one hand. Bend forward slightly at your hips. Lift the dumbbell straight up into your side, bending your arm at the elbow. This is the rowing motion. At the top of the movement, squeeze your back muscles. Next, lower the dumbbell back down to the starting position, using a controlled motion. Switch sides and repeat the exercise with your left arm. Alternate the lift, right arm, then left arm for the designated amount of time in the routine.

## RESISTANCE BAND ROWS

Wrap a resistance band around a pole, tree, bedpost, or other sturdy stationary object, so that it is lined up with the middle of your chest muscles. Stand in front of the object and grab both handles with an overhand grip. Move away from the object until you reach the desired resistance. Keep your chest up, your arms and back straight, and your feet firmly on the floor.

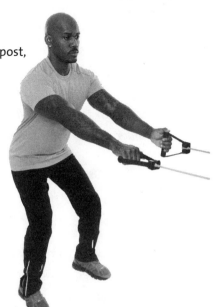

Pull the handles in toward your sides in a rowing motion. Get a good contraction in your back muscles. Return to the starting position, and repeat the exercise for the designated amount of time in the routine.

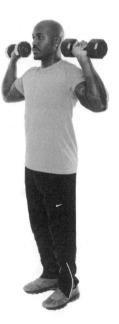

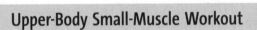

## Upper-Body Small-Muscle Workout

### *SHOULDER PRESS*

*The shoulder press is a great body-shaping exercise for the shoulders and triceps. My male clients like it because it gives them that wide-shouldered masculine look, but my women clients like it too, since it helps tone the back of their upper arms, which tend to get flabby with age. You can perform shoulder presses with dumbbells or resistance bands.*

Use two dumbbells that are 5 to 15 pounds each (for women). Men should be able to use heavier dumbbells, say, 15 to 30 pounds.

Stand with your feet fairly close together, and grasp two dumbbells of equal weight in your hands. Hold them at your shoulders to begin the exercise.

Press your arms straight up so that the weights are overhead.

Repeat this up-and-down motion for the designated amount of time in the routine.

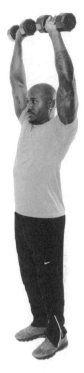

## SIDE LATERALS WITH A RESISTANCE BAND

*This exercise is excellent for shaping the upper arms and shoulders. It is the perfect complement to shoulder presses for an attractive shoulder line that you'll definitely want to show off.*

To begin, place one foot on the center of the band. Grasp the handles in each hand, with your arms out at your sides.

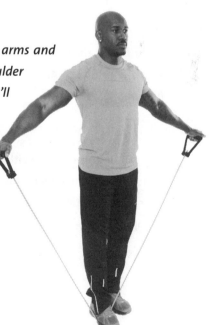

Continue lifting your arms as high as you can. Lower and repeat the motion for the designated amount of time in the routine.

## BICEPS HAMMER CURLS

*Hammer curls work your biceps muscles and your forearms. I like them better than regular curls because they don't significantly strain your wrists. All you need are dumbbells to perform hammer curls.*

You can do this exercise either standing or seated. Grasp two dumbbells of equal weight in your hands and hold them at your sides. Position the dumbbells so that the plate end is facing forward.

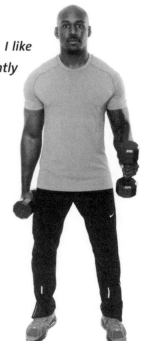

Keep your arms close to your sides. Bend your elbows and slowly curl the left dumbbell up in an arc to a chest-level position. Lower back to the start position.

Bring the right dumbbell up to chest level. Alternate left and right curls for the designated number of minutes in the routine.

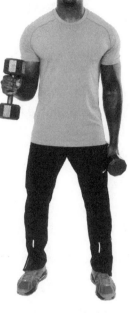

## RESISTANCE BAND HAMMER CURLS

Step on the middle of the resistance band with your right foot. (You can increase the resistance of the band by stepping on the band with both feet and moving your feet farther apart.) Grasp the handles of the band with your palms facing up.

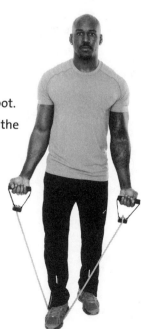

Keep your arms close to your sides. Bend your elbows and slowly curl the handles up in an arc to chest level. Throughout the movement, open your fingers rather than curl them around the handles. This technique makes the exercise more intense.

Slowly lower and repeat.

Continue performing these curls for the designated amount of time in the routine.

## TRICEPS/SHOULDER LIFTS WITH RESISTANCE BANDS

*This exercise primarily works your triceps (at the back of your upper arms), but it also tones the muscles of your shoulders. You won't need any special equipment to perform this move—just your resistance band. It's an intense exercise when you use as much tension as possible, and it delivers great results.*

Stand on the middle section of the band with your right foot slightly forward. Grasp the handles in both hands, palms facing outward.

Press straight upward, getting a good stretch in both triceps. Lock your elbows at the top of the movement. Lower to the starting position and repeat the exercise for 1 minute.

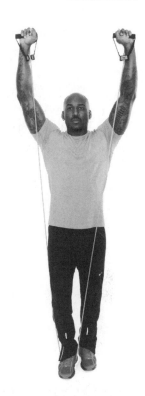

## TRICEPS KICKBACKS WITH DUMBBELLS

*Most people overfocus on working their biceps, to the neglect of their triceps. That's too bad, since the triceps muscle is the largest muscle of the arm, and you don't want it going flabby on you. My workout includes a second triceps exercise—the triceps kickback—to make sure you build strength, tone, and definition in this important muscle. I illustrate how to perform it with dumbbells and resistance bands.*

Grasp a dumbbell in each hand. Bend over slightly, and begin with your right elbow bent and your left arm hanging down.

From this position, press the weight up straight back and lock your elbow. You should feel this move in your triceps.

Next, lower the weight in a controlled fashion. Repeat with the left arm. Alternate right and left arms for the designated amount of time in the routine.

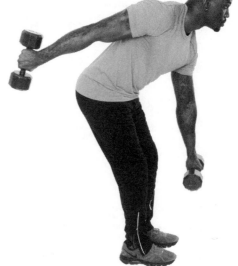

## TRICEPS KICKBACKS WITH A RESISTANCE BAND

Wrap your resistance band around a pole or other sturdy structure. Stand with your legs just slightly apart. Point your toes forward and face the structure. Take the handles in both hands, with your palms facing down. Bend over slightly.

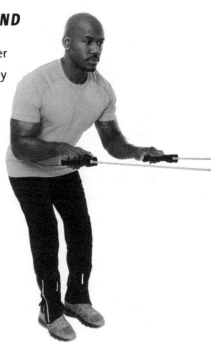

From this position, press the handle straight back and lock your elbow. You should feel this move in your triceps. Next, return the handle to the starting position. Repeat with the left arm. Alternate right and left arms for the designated time in the routine.

# LET'S MOVE IT!

Got it? Those are the exercises you'll be performing. If you want to start burning more fat and losing inches, make sure you've got your workout clothes on, you've laced up your shoes, and you're ready to move.

---

### Dolvett's Dos and Don'ts

*Do* familiarize yourself with the exercise movements before starting the routine; carefully study the exercise descriptions and photos.

*Do* understand that proper form is more important than how much resistance you're using and will lead to *results*.

*Don't* neglect a warm-up prior to working out. For about 5 minutes, do an easy walk or jog while swinging your arms. Another good warm-up is to walk up and down the stairs of your home or simply march in place. When you warm up, you get your muscles ready for the exercises.

*Do* keep your head up (look directly forward at eye level), maintain a straight back, and keep your feet firmly planted on the floor while doing standing movements.

*Do* move the resistance through a full range of motion when you lift.

*Do* focus on smooth, controlled lifting action. Emphasize the eccentric (lowering) phase of the lift. A good rule of thumb to follow is to lower the weight at a rate twice as long as it took to lift it.

*Do* keep your abs tight to help you keep proper body alignment and posture.

*Do* perform your workout in an all-out manner.

*Don't* get dehydrated. Keep your water bottle close by. If you're dehydrated, your strength and energy can drop at least 5 percent. No sodas, either. They are laced with dehydrating caffeine and sugar. Water is your best choice.

*Do* breathe to achieve maximum fitness. While strength training, exhale on the exertion and inhale as you release. During cardio, take natural, consistent breaths in order to deliver oxygen to your working muscles.

*Do* stay focused. Don't watch TV, chat on your cell phone, or do anything that distracts you from working out. Distractions slow you down and adversely affect the quality of your workout.

*Do* cool down after working out. The best cool-down moves are simple stretches. Stretching makes you more flexible and less sore. It also improves circulation to get nutrients to your muscles for toning and repair. So end by stretching all your major muscles in a very simple fashion. For example, lunges to the side will stretch your thighs. Bending over and touching your toes will stretch your hips, back, and hamstrings. Grasping your hands behind your back is a great chest stretch. Hugging yourself is an easy way to stretch your arms and back. Hold each stretch for a few seconds to a point of mild tension, then release; repeat 4 to 5 times. Don't bounce when you stretch. Try to stretch a little farther each time for greater flexibility.

*Do* keep track. Write down an accurate account of your workout progress to ensure accountability, track your progress over time, and keep you motivated. Use the Training Log in the appendix of this book.

*Do* get your doctor's approval prior to beginning an exercise program, especially if you haven't been exercising regularly.

# 7 Go Hard or Go Home: My 48-Minute Workout

The secret to burn-it-off fat loss is an exercise sequence most trainers don't tell you about: *timed circuits* of cardio and strength-training moves. That's what you'll do on this workout. There's no laborious counting or reps or set, just constant movement with minimal rest. You'll perform every exercise, including cardio, for a set number of minutes. This method is truly the best system for burning fat and creating definition in the least amount of workout time.

Warning: This is not exactly circuit training. Let me explain: Traditional circuit-training routines are full-body workouts in which you do consecutive strength-training exercises for every body part in sequential order without resting. Circuit training has its merits, but I'm taking it a few steps further here.

My program adds cardio activity between strength-training exercises, thus keeping your heart rate up and achieving cardiovascular benefits while building muscle. So basically, you start with 6 to 10 minutes of cardio, move to 6 to 10 minutes of lower-body strength exercises, progress to 6 to 10 more minutes of cardio, switch to 6 to 10 minutes of upper-body strength moves, change to 6 to 10 minutes of cardio, then finish with 6 to 10 minutes of small-muscle exercises. The result is a balanced, whole-body workout that builds muscle and aerobic endurance efficiently while burning fat.

You're really getting the best of both worlds too. Cardio burns fat by increasing your body's fat-burning enzymes and circulating more oxygen to your working muscles. That oxygen fans the fat-burning fire. Strength training and resistance exercises add muscle. I can't repeat this enough or say it in too many different ways: The more muscle you have, the faster your metabolism, which means your body is capable of burning fat more efficiently. Various scientific analyses have found that adding just 1 pound of muscle helps burn up to 25,000 more calories a year. That's an automatic 7 pounds of fat scaled off your body, with the addition of just 1 pound of curvy, sexy muscle. Every second of this workout is geared to getting rid of that fat between your skin and muscles and getting you into supersexy shape in the shortest amount of time. When you do this routine faithfully, it will take you into the highest calorie-burning realm—an average of 300 to 500 calories in just 48 minutes!

The proof is in my own experiences. Ever since I introduced my Pure Energy workout, I've seen awesome changes in people in just a few short weeks. Clients who regularly did the workout kept regularly stripping off body fat to reveal amazing muscle definition. I knew that this method of training was the key to becoming super-, if not ultra-, fit.

## I Did It on Dolvett's Program!

I was getting uncomfortably heavy. I was having a hard time zipping up my jeans, and I kept having to buy bigger sizes. I then had to face the music: There was no more denying that I had a weight problem. And I had to do something about it. I made a vow that I would live a healthier, leaner lifestyle.

My biggest problem had always been big portions and second helpings. I would stuff myself like crazy at meals. I'd get so full that I'd have to lie down. Once I started Dolvett's diet, I got a handle on portion control and how much to put on my plate. I started measuring my food and writing down the calories of each portion. At first, this was a bit of a hassle, but now it is second nature. I actually like knowing exactly how many calories I'm eating, because it makes me feel in control of food, rather than feeling like food is in control of me.

After I made the right changes to my diet—more lean proteins, low-sodium foods, fruits, and veggies—I began to see results right away. Every week, I'd lose a few pounds. At the beginning I wasn't exercising, because I hadn't worked out much in the past. But I knew I wouldn't get in real shape unless I worked out. I started the workout, doing 3 sessions a week. It didn't take much time. So I increased the workouts to 5 times a week. That's when I started dropping even more weight, and I could actually see toned muscle on my body. I really got into the whole exercise thing and started mixing it up with yoga and Pilates classes. After 8 months of my new lifestyle, I lost nearly 65 pounds.

I lost 7 pounds the first 2 weeks, and the workout really helped. I added in other activities on my off days: a boot camp class at the gym, paddle boarding, swimming, spinning, and Bikram yoga.

Most of my exercising life, I had been a victim of "all cardio, all the time." I didn't want to waste time with weights, because I just wanted to burn as many calories as possible. But I never seemed to lose weight. At thirty-eight, I feel like I was slowly losing muscle and not addressing it. So lifting weights as part of this workout really made a difference. During the first 2 weeks, I went up in poundages for almost every exercise. I also increased my stamina on the treadmill. I feel like I get better overall results by mixing everything up during each workout, and the fat melted off.

Now that I am at 115 pounds, I feel wonderful. This way of life is a habit for me now. My tips:

- Always make time for exercise and make it a priority. Most activities can be done later, so do your workouts first and then get back to the other stuff.
- Be vocal about your goals and ask for support from your family and friends. They can help you keep your eye on your goals.
- Don't listen to negativity. If someone makes a wisecrack about your progress, tune it out and hang out with people who will support you.

*—Denise S.*

And the proof is also in the science. I'll give you one of many examples. Italian researchers proved in a study of forty middle-aged people that working out using a routine that combined cardio and strength moves trumped a cardio-only routine. The exercisers who performed the combo routine showed the greatest reductions in body weight and fat mass, plus trimmed more inches off their bellies than did the cardio-only exercisers. Strength increased more in the combo group too. What you're about to do really works wonders on the body.

Do you already do some exercise? That's great, and if you're someone who endures well at cardio, but you have no real muscle strength or tone, this workout will bring your strength up to par with your cardiovascular ability. Or if you're strong but you don't do well with cardio, this workout will condition your heart and lungs so that you're more aerobically fit.

This workout will feel intense for everyone. But don't worry, your exhaustion will be overtaken by the fun you'll have while doing it. At the end of each workout, you'll be a sweaty, panting heap of a body. A week or two into this workout, your body will start feeling and looking great. Keep it up and you'll never stay fat at this rate. Oh, wait—that's the point, isn't it?

Because this is an intense, fast-moving workout, select light to moderate weights based on your fitness level. I recommend that women use weights between 5 and 15 pounds and men use weights between 15 and 30 pounds. But that's just for starters. After a couple of weeks, I want you to increase the amount of weight you're using in this routine. You've got to progressively increase your poundages to progressively get more results. Using the same poundage workout after workout will result in stagnation, and I want you to keep getting better, stronger, and more fit, every single workout.

This is a workout you can do in the convenience of your own home. Make sure you have enough space and the room is well ventilated. Keep your water bottle handy too. Put on your favorite music, and get ready to jam and sweat. I predict this workout will rival anything you've ever done.

## Dolvett's Dos and Don'ts

*Do* be accountable. Put a calendar on your refrigerator and attach a red marker and a green marker to the calendar. For any day you've had a good day—you've exercised for 48 minutes or more, you've eaten the right foods, you've made good choices all day long, taken good care of yourself—mark a green line on that date. Redline the days you ditched your workout, overate, or slipped into some bad habits like smoking or drinking too much. Every time you get into your refrigerator, that calendar's looking at you. Trust me, you want to be seeing more green lines than red ones.

*Do* set exercise mini-goals. Small steps get you where you want to be. So set some mini-challenges for exercising. Some examples: *I will increase my cardio this week. I will increase my strength-training minutes. I will try one new fun activity this week. I will increase my poundage and resistances this week.* When you get down to specific, manageable challenges, you will succeed, and that success builds momentum. Next thing you know, you're in better shape than you've ever been in.

*Do* go on the attack. First thing after you wake up in the morning, attack your physique. Roll out of bed and hit the floor. Do my 48-minute routine and give your body a quick explosion of muscle development. And then go brush your teeth!

*Do* buddy up. Make a plan with friends or co-workers to do some workouts together. On your cardio day, for example, just go for a walk together. Next week, turn that walk into a light jog. The week after that, turn that light jog into a run. If you start a community in exercise, the likelihood of your being successful will be greater.

*Do* adopt a "Get It Done" attitude. Tell yourself: *I can finish this in 48 minutes. I can do this. This is the perfect workout to define my muscles and get ready for bathing suit season. I love working out.*

*Don't* let time get in the way. Simply find time; better yet, make time! Set your alarm clock an hour earlier than normal. Wake up and hit the gym early, or do your home workout right away. This schedule will give you lots of energy and focus throughout your day. Remember, this is just a 48-minute workout, and even the busiest person can take that much time for exercise.

*Don't* skip workouts on the road or while working late. Fit in sweat sessions whenever possible. You're stuck in a hotel room or working late in your office cubicle. Don't let these constraints stop you. Keep your resistance bands with you so you can do my resistance exercises. Use the hotel or office chair. Grab it and do some dips. Let the edge of the chair be the ending point for your squats. Put your feet on the chair and do push-ups. Another idea if you're on vacation: Wake up every morning with a yoga routine or a run. Early-morning workouts energize your day and give you that toned, lean feeling you can take with you all day.

*Do* play music while working out. Music is motivating, so crank up your favorite playlist and move. Mine is hip-hop. I work out to it every day.

# DAY 1 ROUTINE

## First Cardio Timed Sequence

10 minutes of cardio: Walk or jog on the treadmill on an incline. Start at a speed of 3.5 miles per hour and set the treadmill at a level 6 incline. *Every 2 minutes, increase your incline by a few numbers; for example, from 3 to 5, or higher.* If you don't have a treadmill, march or run in place for 10 minutes.

## Lower-Body Timed Sequence: 10 Minutes of Strength Training

Squats or Resistance Band Squats:
Perform the exercise for 2 minutes.

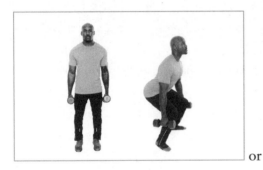 or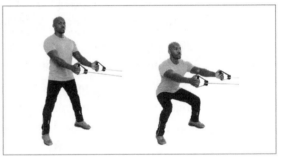

Forward Lunge or Resistance Band Lunge:
Perform the exercise for 2 minutes.

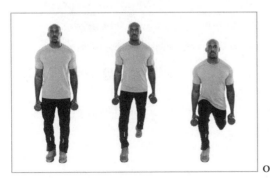 or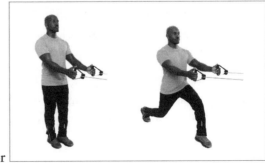

Backward Lunge: Perform the exercise for 2 minutes.

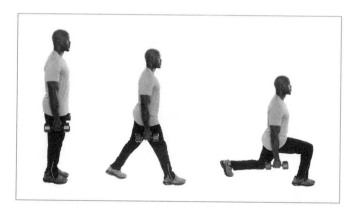

Dead Lifts: Perform the exercise for 2 minutes.

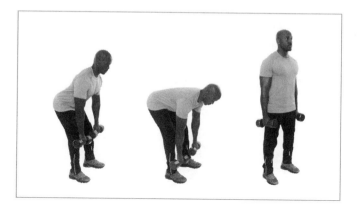

Sumo Squats: Perform the exercise for 1 minute.

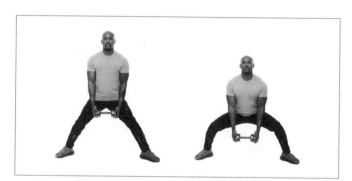

Hamstring Lifts: Perform the exercise for 1 minute.

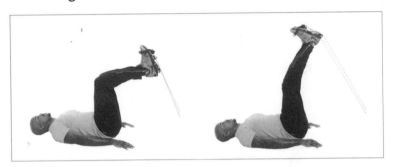

## Second Cardio Timed Sequence

8 minutes of cardio: Jump rope, run up and down stairs, or use home cardio equipment, if available.

## Upper-Body Large-Muscle Timed Sequence: 8 Minutes of Strength Training

Alternate Push-ups and Planks for 2 minutes.

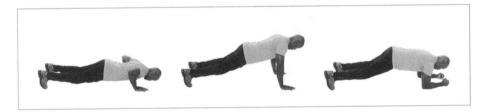

Chest Butterfly Press on Mat or Butterfly Press with a Resistance Band: Perform the exercise for 2 minutes.

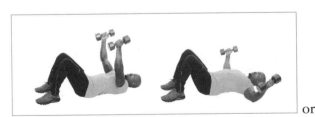  or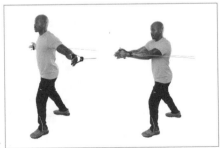

Dumbbell Chest Press: Perform the exercise for 2 minutes.

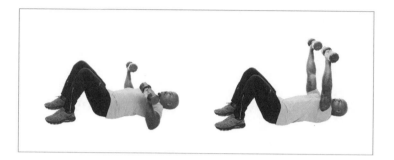

Dumbbell Pullover: Perform the exercise for 1 minute.

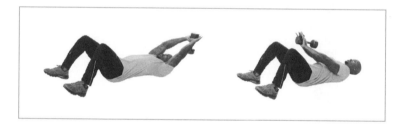

Dumbbell Rows or Resistance Band Rows: Perform the exercise for 1 minute.

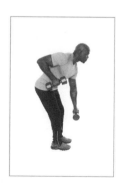 or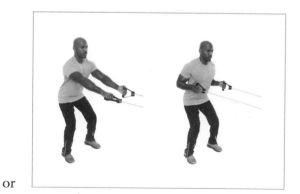

## Third Cardio Timed Sequence

6 minutes of cardio: Jump rope, run up and down stairs, or use home cardio equipment, if available.

## Upper-Body Small-Muscle Timed Sequence: 6 Minutes of Strength Training

Shoulder Press: Perform the exercise for 1 minute.

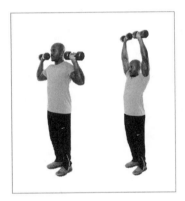

Side Laterals with a Resistance Band:
Perform the exercise for 1 minute.

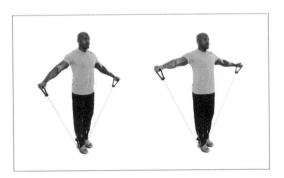

Biceps Hammer Curls or Resistance Band Hammer Curls:
Perform the exercise for 2 minutes.

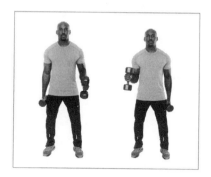 or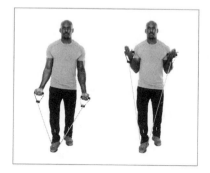

Triceps Kickbacks with Dumbbells or a Resistance Band:
Perform the exercise for 2 minutes.

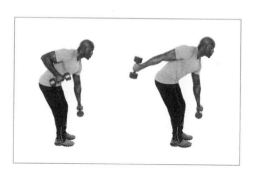 or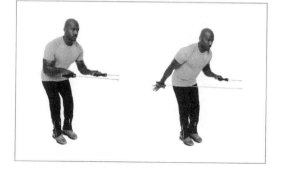

# DAY 2 ROUTINE

Repeat the entire Day 1 routine.

# DAY 3 ROUTINE

## First Cardio Timed Sequence

6 minutes of cardio: Walk or jog on the treadmill on an incline. Start at a speed of 3.5 miles per hour and set the treadmill at a level 6 incline. *Every 2 minutes, increase your incline by a few numbers; for example, from 3 to 5, or higher.* If you don't have a treadmill, march or run in place for 6 minutes.

## Lower-Body Timed Sequence: 6 Minutes of Strength Training

Squats or Resistance Band Squats: Perform the exercise for 2 minutes.

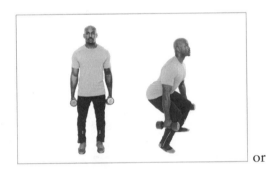 or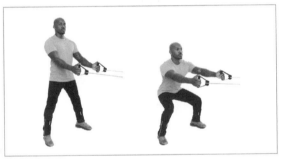

Forward Lunge or Resistance Band Lunge: Perform the exercise for 2 minutes.

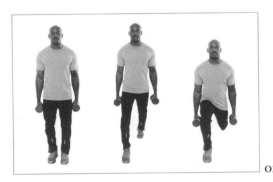 or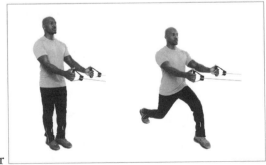

Dead Lifts: Perform the exercise for 2 minutes.

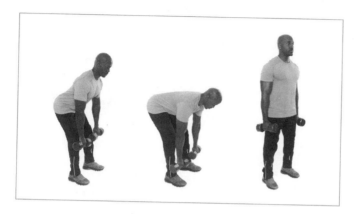

## Second Cardio Timed Sequence

8 minutes of cardio: Jump rope, run up and down stairs, or use home cardio equipment, if available.

## Upper-Body Large-Muscle Timed Sequence: 8 Minutes of Strength Training

Alternate Push-ups and Planks for 1 minute.

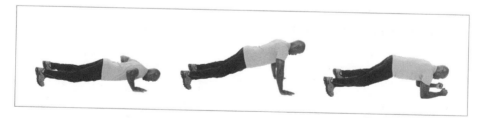

Chest Butterfly Press on Mat or Butterfly Press with a
Resistance Band: Perform the exercise for 2 minutes.

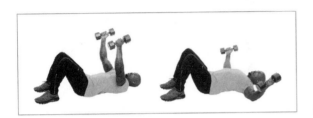 or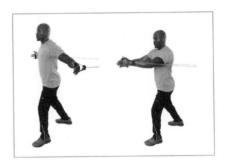

Dumbbell Chest Press: Perform the exercise for 2 minutes.

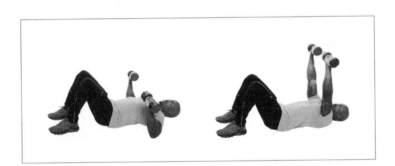

Dumbbell Pullover: Perform the exercise for 1 minute.

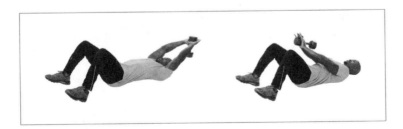

Dumbbell Rows or Resistance Band Rows:
Perform the exercise for 2 minutes.

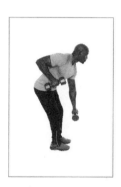 or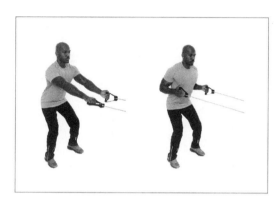

## Third Cardio Timed Sequence

10 minutes of cardio: Walk or jog on the treadmill on an incline. Start at a speed of 3.5 miles per hour and set the treadmill at a level 6 incline. *Every 2 minutes, increase your incline by a few numbers; for example, from 3 to 5, or higher.* If you don't have a treadmill, march or run in place for 10 minutes.

## Upper-Body Small-Muscle Timed Sequence: 10 Minutes of Strength Training

Shoulder Press: Perform the exercise for 2 minutes.

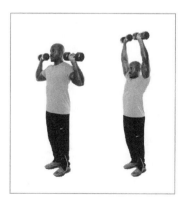

Side Laterals with a Resistance Band:
Perform the exercise for 2 minutes.

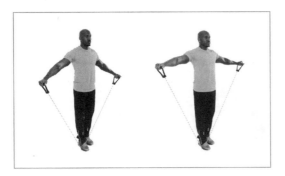

Biceps Hammer Curls or Resistance Band Hammer Curls:
Perform the exercise for 2 minutes.

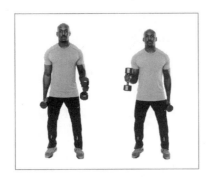 or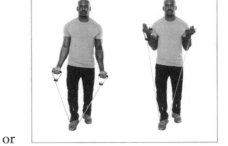

Triceps/Shoulder Lifts with a Resistance Band:
Perform the exercise for 2 minutes.

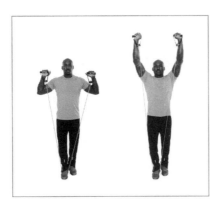

Triceps Kickbacks with Dumbbells or a Resistance Band:
Perform the exercise for 2 minutes.

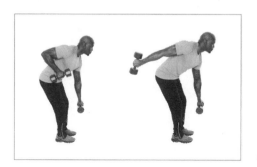 or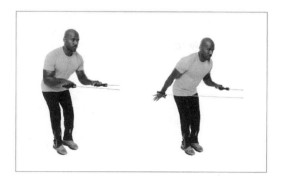

## DAY 4 ROUTINE

Repeat the entire Day 3 routine.

## DAY 5 ROUTINE

*Rest*: No workout! Everyone should have a day of rest. It helps the body recover and keeps your life in balance.

## DAY 6 ROUTINE

Perform at least 60 minutes of any cardio activity you enjoy.

## DAY 7 FUN ROUTINE

Enjoy at least 60 minutes of active fun. Incidentally, you can swap day 6 and day 7, depending on your schedule and preference. My own "fun day" is crazy. There's nothing I don't do. I involve everything from yoga to Zumba to hiking to Pilates to sports in my routine. You have to pick exciting things along the way. Are you taking a Zumba or Pilates class? What about challenging yourself to a warrior dash with your friends? Don't limit yourself to just going to the gym, and don't make it robotic. Make it fun! I've listed some additional ideas for you in the next box.

| 50 Ways to Leave Your Blubber ||
| Activities | Approximate Calories Burned in 1 Hour |
| --- | --- |
| Aerobic dance | 352 |
| Archery | 246 |
| Badminton | 317 |
| Ballet | 317 |
| Baseball | 352 |
| Basketball | 422 |
| Belly dancing | 303 |
| Biking | 563 |
| Bowling | 211 |
| Boxing, sparring | 633 |
| Canoeing | 493 |
| Climbing | 528 |
| Cross-country skiing | 563 |
| Dancing | 387 |
| Fencing | 422 |
| Football, touch | 563 |
| Gardening | 281 |
| Golf, walking and carrying clubs | 317 |
| Handball | 844 |
| Hiking | 422 |
| Horseback riding | 381 |
| Ice-skating | 493 |
| Jazzercise | 422 |
| Kayaking | 352 |

| | |
|---|---|
| Martial arts | 704 |
| Motorcycle riding | 176 |
| Mountain biking | 598 |
| Pilates | 168 |
| Racquetball | 493 |
| Rollerblading | 844 |
| Rollerskating | 387 |
| Rowboating | 844 |
| Scuba diving | 493 |
| Skateboarding | 352 |
| Snorkeling | 352 |
| Snowshoeing | 563 |
| Snow skiing | 422 |
| Softball | 352 |
| Squash | 844 |
| Surfing | 211 |
| Swimming | 493 |
| Table tennis | 281 |
| Tennis | 493 |
| Vigorous play with your kids | 352 |
| Volleyball | 211 |
| Water aerobics | 281 |
| Wii sports games | 354 |
| Windsurfing | 211 |
| Yoga | 281 |
| Zumba, or any Latin fusion workout | 500 |

*Calculations are based on research data from* Medicine and Science in Sports and Exercise, *the official journal of the American College of Sports Medicine.*

---

## AFFIRM TO GET FIRM: VISUALIZATION

See yourself as an exerciser or athlete. Visualize clearly and vividly your life as an active person—as if it has already taken place. You will activate all kinds of subconscious activity to make your vision come true. I've worked with a lot of people, men and women, who wondered whether they could ever become active on a regular basis. When I introduce them to strength training, which is something that requires very little athletic skill, most folks take to it right away. It makes them feel like athletes and see themselves that way, and it helps them forge a stronger identity as exercisers. They view themselves as athletes, and their newly active lifestyles become part of who they are.

---

# HOW TO PROGRESS

I'm going to push you now and make you push yourself. On *The Biggest Loser*, I'm a bit of a screamer, but it's only because I'm passionate about what I do. I want people—including you—to find their inner athlete, and that's not going to come out by me whispering. It never has and never will. Granted, I can't be standing next to you, screaming at you to push, but I want you to go hard here or go home. Get passionate about this and stay passionate.

## Week 2

One way to tap into that passion is to challenge yourself to do more each week. For example, this week you started out with 48-minute workouts. In your second week, I want you to pick up the pace. Go for longer cardio sequences, such as 12 to 15 minutes, and do the strength exercises for 3 minutes each.

From there, make another adjustment in training that will speed up your progress. Challenge yourself to use more weight in each movement. Use as heavy a resistance as you can handle for 6 to 8 reps. Pay attention to good form, but using more weight is what will help your muscles develop and grow.

## Week 3

In your third week, increase your cardio speed and your incline level. Continue to increase your resistances on strength-training moves.

At the end of your third week of training, you'll have laid the foundation of a strong, shapely physique, and your health and mental state should be improving as well. And by the end of this week, you'll see some noticeable changes in your physique. Seeing visible changes is one of the most motivating forces that'll drive you to maintain your exercise program. Keep it up!

## Beyond Week 3

At this point, it's time to make some more large-scale changes in your workout. One of the easiest things to do is to increase your exercise time. When you're ready and even more pumped, turn this routine into 90 minutes of pure, heart-pounding, fat-burning craziness. Do your cardio sequences for 15 minutes each and your exercises for 3 to 5 minutes each. I want you to love working out as much as I do, and feel it as a release, like I do. To help you stay on track and increase your progress, I've included a Training Log in the appendix. Use it and congratulate yourself on the gains you're making every single week.

You should stick with a particular workout for 3 to 4 weeks to allow your body to grow as demands are placed upon it, but eventually your muscles will adapt to a specific routine. Experiment with some different exercises and do them in your routine. The process of continual change keeps your muscles confused—and constantly stimulated.

There is a lot of variety in what you can try, because you can do a given movement any number of ways: with a barbell, dumbbells, or resistance bands. People switch up their routines because they've learned what works best for them and what makes their body respond. You will, too, as you learn more about your body. After a while, you'll develop an instinctive sense as to how to manipulate the training variables, and you'll know when it's time to change things up.

## AFFIRM TO GET FIRM: STOP THE EXCUSES

Your mind can trip you up. Some days, you might hear messages like, *I don't feel like working out today. I'll do it tomorrow. I'll make up for today by doing twice as much tomorrow.* And on and on. Don't give in to this nonsense. Tell your mind to get out of your body's way. Talk back: *I've got work to do, mind. Sorry, not today.* Say positive things to yourself at your weakest hour, and stop talking yourself out of the possible.

# Part Three

*The 3-1-2-1 Maintenance Plan*

# 8 The 3-1-2-1 Maintenance Diet: Lean Toward Clean

You've spent a productive length of time on my plan, and I trust you've reached your ideal weight. Your hard work has paid some positive dividends. You love the way you look in the mirror. No longer do you have to suck in fast to put on your skirt or pants. No longer do you have to respond to questions like "What's up?" with "Just my weight and cholesterol." And those running shoes of yours are finally out of hibernation. You've gotten to a healthy mind-set, and you're on the right track to success. That doesn't mean your work, or mine, is done, though. I want to continue to motivate, inspire, and encourage you to understand that you have the power to continue this new lifestyle and keep your weight off. I don't want your fat to find its way back after being lost, and neither do you, unless you want a verbal kick in the butt from me.

As a personal trainer, I've worked with hundreds of people who have maintained their new ideal weight for many years. One of the biggest success factors is diet. Here I want to give you the maintenance version of my 3-1-2-1 Diet to keep you on track.

## A DIET FOR YOUR LIFETIME

Bad news: You can't go back to your old eating habits. You do have to eat right on your noncheat days for the rest of your life to stay in shape. In my experience with "successful losers," I've observed that people who keep their weight off stick to the same meal plans that helped them lose weight in the first place. That means making proper choices most days of the week: lean proteins, greens, and colorful fruits and vegetables—and staying away from heavy, white starches and corn. In fact, I always advise people to eat like they're living on an island and consuming natural foods indigenous to island life: nuts, fruits, grains, fresh vegetables, and fish. If you're conscious about doing this FIVE days a week, you'll be eating a balanced diet that will keep you lean.

Good news: The 3-1-2-1 Diet is definitely sustainable for a lifetime. You can enjoy your favorite foods, without being too rigid, and you can eat clean the rest of the time. This approach is the best maintenance formula you'll ever find. To maintain your weight loss, lean toward clean, but allow yourself a little more freedom. That's what the 3-1-2-1 Maintenance Diet does. Here's what I mean:

*Modifying the 3-1-2-1 Diet.* On maintenance, you'll continue to stick to the principles of the 3-1-2-1 Diet. Eat the same healthy foods you ate while on my plan, and enjoy 2 cheat days weekly. Some dietary indiscretions here and there will not undo all your hard work, so give yourself permission to enjoy your favorite foods once in a while.

*Calories Still Count.* Be aware of how calories work. I never downplay calories. They measure an important energy issue with your body, and that has to do with how the body handles the balance between how much you eat and how much you burn. If you eat more calories than your body burns off (through activity, breathing, and general movement), then your body packs the excess away as body fat. Conversely, if you burn off more calories than you consume, then your body taps into stored fat for energy. In a nutshell, that's how you lose weight. Thus, balancing calorie intake with caloric burn off has everything to do with whether you gain weight, lose weight, or maintain weight. This makes a prescription for keeping weight off pretty simple. You need to know how many calories you can eat daily to maintain your new, thinner weight.

The trick, of course, is figuring out how many calories are enough. There are a lot of complicated math formulas you can do, or you can undergo tests at research centers. I've got an easier method, however, and you don't have to be a math whiz to figure this out. Just grab a calculator and/or a pen and paper. All you need to know is your present weight in pounds.

I don't care how math challenged you are; you can do these calculations: Take your new, ideal body weight in pounds and multiply it by 12 if you're a woman and by 13 if you're a man. The number at which you'll arrive is your daily maintenance caloric intake—the number of calories that will keep you at your ideal weight. Thus, a 130-pound woman needs to eat 1,560 calories daily to maintain her weight; a 175-pound man, 2,275.

These numbers assume that you're exercising at least 4 times a week for 48 minutes (as my workout lays out) to 1 hour each session. A caveat: These numbers are estimations; every person is different. You may be off by 100 or 200 calories a day. If you find you're gaining weight, shave calories off your maintenance intake. It's all about tweaking.

I believe that a calorie is a calorie is a calorie—whether you're eating your favorite dessert, having Thanksgiving dinner, or socializing at a party with a plate full of nachos and *queso*. If you eat something, it has calories. Here's the difference: Some calories are nutritious and others aren't. On my maintenance plan, I emphasize mostly nutritious calories—healthy foods that help your body stay at its ideal weight.

Ultimately, keeping your ideal weight all comes down to numbers—calories in, calories out—and finding the right balance to stay at your ideal weight permanently. I can't say it too many times or explain it any other way: Tilt your calories toward the high side and the pounds will pile on, but tilt them the other way, even slightly, and you'll keep your weight off.

## AFFIRM TO GET FIRM: DARE TO BE DIFFERENT

I've encouraged my *Biggest Loser* teams with these words: Don't be another one. Be the OTHER one. That's the person who keeps his or her weight off and is not just another statistic in the pile of people who regain all those pounds. That's the person who defies the naysayers who say you can't lose weight or get in shape or run a marathon. That's the person who says no to drugs, alcohol abuse, and junk-food binges. Really successful people, people who outpace the pack in life, have one distinguishing characteristic: They stand out from the crowd in positive ways.
So dare to be different and you will be on the road to becoming the best person you can be, in the best shape you can obtain.

# FOLLOWING THE 3-1-2-1 MAINTENANCE DIET

I've created four sample weekly menus to show you how the 3-1-2-1 Maintenance Diet works. Basically, you'll be following the same pattern as you did on the weight-loss diet, but like this: 3 days of clean maintenance eating, 1 day of cheat maintenance eating, 2 days of clean maintenance eating, and 1 day of cheat maintenance eating.

Some important guidelines:

- Increase your calories in maintenance by increasing the size of your Smart Proteins by an ounce or two; by eating an extra portion of your Smart Carbs; by increasing your snack choices; or all of the above.
- Emphasize the healthiest calories possible: lean proteins, good carbs, and lots of vegetables and fruits.
- Lean toward low-fat, high-fiber products.
- Choose gluten-free foods whenever possible.
- Continue to use Dolvett's Dish to plan your meals: 1 Smart Protein, 1 Smart Fiber, and 1 Smart Carb on your plate at each main meal. Portion control is even more important to weight maintenance. Keep your portions as close to my suggested sizes as possible. When you boil up a pot of brown rice, for example, you can't eat the whole batch and still keep your weight under control. Use measuring cups and spoons to help you manage portions—no eyeballing. I've often suggested to clients that they serve their meals on salad plates because they're smaller than dinner plates. This technique helps you keep portions within the correct range.
- Always eat slowly. Put your utensils down between bites, and chew your food thoroughly. It takes around 20 minutes for your brain to tell your stomach that it's full, so stretch your meals out.
- Watch your fats. You'll need to include some healthy fats in your diet. They are vital for a speedy metabolism, but bad fats will slow it down. Bad fats are saturated fats such as butter, animal fat, cream, and trans fats. These fats raise cholesterol, which, as well as being bad for your heart, makes the blood sticky so it doesn't flow well through the body. This stops your bodily processes—including your metabolism—from working efficiently. Continue to eat olive oil, flaxseed

oil, and light salad dressings—in moderation. On maintenance, you can also eat trans-fat-free margarine in tiny amounts. Remember too: Fats are condiments on my plan.

■ Drink water throughout the day. If you've heard this advice once, you've heard it a million times. Water is the true secret ingredient for keeping weight off. Not only does it prevent fluid retention and bloat, but it's also a natural appetite suppressant and helps your body burn stored fat. You need to drink half of your body weight (in ounces) in water a day, more if you exercise.

■ On cheat days, add no more than 300 calories to your day's intake.

■ Eat frequently through the day to keep your burn rate up. Time your snacks so that your body is never waiting longer than 2 to 3 hours for food.

■ Do not force-feed yourself. Just because your daily maintenance calories tally up to 1,600 or 1,800, that doesn't mean you must eat all those calories. For weeks now, you've been eating a calorie-controlled diet, with smaller portions, and your stomach may have shrunk as a result. Yes, I believe your stomach does shrink somewhat when you diet. Your stomach is made up of layers of muscles, all capable of contracting or stretching. When there is very little inside, the muscles contract and the stomach gets smaller. Also, your stomach shrinks mentally, in a manner of speaking. You've gotten used to smaller portions and lower caloric intake, meaning that you've formed new eating habits. And that's a mental process. You're physically and mentally used to eating less food, so consume your allotted maintenance only when you feel hungry.

## THE 3-1-2-1 MAINTENANCE DIET MENUS

Here are sample menus for four different levels of caloric intake: 1,600 calories a day, 1,800 calories a day, 2,000 calories a day, and 2,300 calories a day. To my women readers: Most of you will follow the 1,600-calories-a-day maintenance plan. If you find you're gaining weight on this program, scale back your daily calories to 1,400 or 1,500 calories a day. You can do this by subtracting a Smart Carb or two or by eating smaller portions of Smart Proteins.

Guys: You'll be following the 1,800-, 2,000-, or 2,300-calories-a-day program, depending on what the math calculations revealed about what it takes to maintain your

## I DID IT ON DOLVETT'S PROGRAM!

Several years ago, I was in a car accident that caused major knee and lower-back pain. I could not exercise for many months. Pounds started to pile on, and my health was in jeopardy. I couldn't do anything because of the pain, and I felt very depressed. I started getting chiropractic care, and that helped me heal. I still had some residual pain, but I felt ready to tackle my weight.

I started the 3-1-2-1 Diet, and with it, the exercise program (which I had to start very slowly at first, only 3 times a week). Even so, I quickly felt like I was getting stronger, physically and mentally. I wanted to explore some other workouts too, as Dolvett suggests, so I signed up for martial arts. It really helped me focus—not to mention that my legs and butt got in great shape too.

I found the diet to be very livable. I gradually lost weight, about 3 pounds a week at first. I shed 25 pounds in 3 months. To celebrate, I went on a shopping spree to buy some new clothes. I started getting lots of compliments on my new shape, and this boosted my self-esteem. I turned 45 last month, and I feel like I'm in the best shape of my life. Best of all, I've kept my weight off for 3 years.

My tips:

- Weigh yourself several times a week. This helps me stay aware of my weight. Sometimes it's not pretty, but frequent weighing forces me to be honest with myself, so I step on the scale often.
- Give yourself a "grace weight." For me, that's 5 pounds above my goal weight. When I hit that limit, I get back to the basic plan: making proper food choices, measuring portions, counting calories, and sticking to my exercise plan.
- Always exercise harder on cheat days. You're eating more calories on cheat days, so why not burn more of them? I make it a point to work out longer and harder on cheat days to burn those extra 300 or more calories I'm eating. For example, I like to jog on a treadmill or exercise on an elliptical trainer that tracks my caloric burn. I don't stop until I've expended 300 calories or more.

*—Courtney F.*

weight. If you find you're gaining weight on any of these plans, cut back on your calories, or follow one of the lower-calorie maintenance plans.

There are 7 sample days in each plan. These menus give you examples of how to eat to maintain your weight, based on your maintenance calories. You can follow these exactly or create your own based on your calorie needs.

One more point: I've incorporated cheat days into each of these sample menus. On maintenance you may not feel like cheating twice a week. If so, then don't! Save your cheating for special occasions or weekends.

## 7-Day Meal Plan: 1,600 Calories

### Day 1

**Breakfast**

1 cup of pineapple chunks, fresh or canned in juice
1 cup of low-fat cottage cheese
5 whole wheat crackers

**Snack**

1 medium orange

**Lunch**

Peanut butter and jelly sandwich: 2 slices of multigrain, gluten-free bread
spread with 2 tablespoons of peanut butter and 1 tablespoon of all-fruit spread
or sugar-free jelly
1 medium apple

**Snack**

Handful of almonds or walnuts

### Dinner

5-ounce boneless skinless chicken breast, broiled or grilled

1 medium baked sweet potato, topped with 1 teaspoon of trans-fat-free
  margarine

Large tossed salad: 2 cups of tossed mixed greens topped with 1 small tomato
  (chopped) and drizzled with 2 tablespoons of light salad dressing

*Total Calories: 1,672*

## Day 2

### Breakfast

2 scrambled eggs topped with 1 tablespoon of shredded cheddar cheese and
  2 tablespoons of salsa

1 slice of toasted rye bread, topped with 1 teaspoon of trans-fat-free
  margarine

1 cup of almond milk

### Snack

*Tropical Delight* smoothie, page 104

### Lunch

Turkey sandwich: 2 slices of multigrain, gluten-free bread with 3 slices of fat-free
  turkey ham, 1 slice of Swiss cheese, 2 lettuce leaves, 2 slices of tomato, and
  1 tablespoon of dark mustard

1 medium pear

### Snack

½ cup of low-fat frozen yogurt (your favorite flavor)

### Dinner

Large fillet of salmon, grilled
½ cup of cooked brown rice
1 cup of boiled or steamed broccoli

**Total Calories: 1,673**

## Day 3

### Breakfast

1 cup of high-fiber cereal (such as Fiber One or All-Bran)
1 cup of fresh sliced strawberries
1 cup of almond milk

### Snack

Handful of almonds or walnuts

### Lunch

1 medium (6") whole wheat pita bread pocket, served with ½ cup of hummus
1 cup of grape or cherry tomatoes

### Snack

1 medium apple

### Dinner

Hamburger on a hamburger bun, topped with 1 slice of cheddar cheese and
    1 tablespoon of mustard
*Sweet Potato Fries*, page 123

**Total Calories: 1,557**

## Day 4 (Maintenance Cheat Day)

### Breakfast

1 cup of cooked oatmeal, topped with 2 tablespoons of chopped walnuts
1 cup of fresh blueberries
1 cup of almond milk

### Snack

Handful of almonds

### Lunch

1 cup of macaroni and cheese
Tossed green salad with 2 tablespoons of light salad dressing

### Snack

1 medium peach

### Dinner

*Barbecue restaurant dinner:*
1 serving of barbecued ribs
1 serving of creamy coleslaw
1 serving of baked beans

*Total Calories: 1,936*

### Restaurant Calorie Red Alert!

A dinner like this can add up to 600 calories or more, depending on the restaurant. Be familiar with meal calories at restaurants before you go.

## Day 5

*Breakfast*

1 cup of oatmeal topped with 2 tablespoons of chopped walnuts and sweetened with 1 tablespoon of honey

2 hard-boiled eggs

½ grapefruit

*Snack*

*Rise and Grind Smoothie*, page 104

*Lunch*

*Smart Tuna Salad*, page 112

1 slice of multigrain, gluten-free bread

1 cup of fresh blueberries

*Snack*

1 cup of low-fat yogurt (your favorite flavor)

*Dinner*

10 large shrimp, grilled

1 cup of steamed asparagus, topped with 1 teaspoon of trans-fat-free margarine

1 cup of brown rice

*Total Calories: 1,678*

## Day 6

*Breakfast*

2 scrambled eggs made with a handful of fresh spinach and 3 tablespoons of
    chopped tomato
2 slices of multigrain, gluten-free toast

*Snack*

1 medium pear
1 cup of almond milk

*Lunch*

Turkey sandwich: 2 slices of multigrain, gluten-free bread with 3 slices of fat-free
    turkey ham, 1 slice of Swiss cheese, 2 lettuce leaves, 2 slices of tomato, and
    1 tablespoon of dark mustard
1 medium apple

*Snack*

*Yogurt Berry Shake*, page 105

*Dinner*

Large fillet of tilapia, baked or broiled
1 cup of steamed mixed vegetables
½ cup of cooked quinoa

*Total Calories: 1,664*

## Day 7 (Maintenance Cheat Day)

### Breakfast

Two whole-grain toaster waffles, topped with 1 cup of berries, 2 teaspoons of
  trans-fat-free margarine, and 1 tablespoon of sugar-free maple syrup
1 cup of almond milk

### Snack

*A+ Smoothie*, page 105

### Lunch

1 turkey hot dog with mustard on a whole wheat hot dog roll
1 cup of sliced red bell peppers

### Snack

1 medium apple

### Dinner

*Italian dinner:*
1 serving of lasagna
Tossed mixed green salad with 1 tablespoon of Italian dressing
1 bread stick
2 glasses (5 ounces each) of red wine

*Total Calories: 1,842*

---

### Restaurant Calorie Red Alert!

An Italian dinner like this can add up to 700 calories or more, depending on the restaurant. Be familiar with meal calories at restaurants before you go. At some Italian restaurants, a serving size of lasagna can have as many as 850 calories.

---

# 7-DAY MEAL PLAN: 1,800 CALORIES

## Day 1

*Breakfast*

2 lean turkey sausage links

1 scrambled egg

2 slices of multigrain, gluten-free toast with 1 teaspoon of trans-fat-free margarine

½ grapefruit

*Snack*

*Rise and Grind Smoothie*, page 104

*Lunch*

1 chicken breast, grilled or baked

1 medium sweet potato

1 medium apple

*Snack*

Handful of almonds or walnuts

*Dinner*

Large pork chop, broiled or grilled

Pasta salad made with 1 cup of cooked whole wheat or gluten-free pasta,
    1 tablespoon of chopped onion, 2 tablespoons of chopped red bell pepper,
    Italian seasonings to taste, and 1 teaspoon of olive oil

1 cup of cooked, drained spinach topped with 1 teaspoon of trans-fat-free
    margarine

*Total Calories: 1,868*

## Day 2

*Breakfast*

1 cup of oatmeal

1 cup of almond milk

1 cup of orange juice

*Snack*

1 cup of low-fat yogurt (your favorite flavor)

1 medium apple

*Lunch*

Ham sandwich: 2 slices of multigrain, gluten-free bread with 3 slices of
    fat-free ham, 1 slice of Swiss cheese, 2 lettuce leaves, 2 slices of tomato,
    and 1 tablespoon of dark mustard or 1 tablespoon of mashed avocado

*Snack*

1 protein bar (with at least 20 grams of protein)

### Dinner

5-ounce sirloin steak, grilled
1 cup of brown rice
Tossed green salad with 2 tablespoons of light salad dressing

*Total Calories: 1,874*

## Day 3

### Breakfast

Omelet made with 2 eggs, diced fat-free ham (1 slice) and ½ cup of sliced mushrooms
2 slices of whole wheat toast with 1 teaspoon of trans-fat-free margarine
1 cup of fresh blueberries or strawberries

### Snack

*A+ Smoothie,* page 105

### Lunch

*Chicken Cobb Salad,* page 109
1 bread stick

### Snack

1 cup of low-fat yogurt (your favorite flavor)

### Dinner

Large fillet of salmon, baked or broiled
1 cup of steamed mixed vegetables
½ cup of brown rice

*Total Calories: 1,799*

## Day 4 (Maintenance Cheat Day)

*Breakfast*

3 pancakes with 1 tablespoon of sugar-free maple syrup
2 slices of turkey bacon
1 cup of sliced strawberries

*Snack*

1 medium apple

*Lunch*

*Fast-food lunch:*
Grilled chicken sandwich

### Restaurant Calorie Red Alert!

A healthy fast-food choice like a grilled chicken sandwich contains between 300 and 400 calories. It's easy to find the calorie counts of fast foods; just log on to the companies' websites for calorie information.

*Snack*

Chocolate candy bar

### Dinner

*Mexican dinner:*
2 beef or chicken fajitas
1 serving of Mexican rice or beans
1 margarita

**Total Calories: 2,034**

---

### Restaurant Calorie Red Alert!

A Mexican dinner like this can add up to 500 calories or more, depending on the restaurant. When you order something like a margarita, be aware that depending on the recipe and the size of the drink, it can be loaded with calories. A small margarita starts at 150 calories per drink, on average. Larger margaritas can be much higher.

## Day 5

### Breakfast

1 cup of oatmeal sweetened with 1 tablespoon of honey
1 cup of fresh blueberries
1 cup of almond milk

### Snack

1 cup of yogurt (your favorite flavor)

*Lunch*

1 cup of vegetable soup

1 tossed green salad with a variety of salad vegetables (bell peppers, cherry tomatoes, cucumber slices, 2 tablespoons of chopped onion) topped with 3 slices of fat-free ham (chopped) and drizzled with 2 tablespoons of light salad dressing

5 whole wheat crackers

1 medium pear

*Snack*

1 protein bar (with at least 20 grams of protein)

*Dinner*

1 large pork chop, grilled or broiled

1 cup of steamed broccoli

1 whole wheat roll

*Total Calories: 1,834*

## Day 6

*Breakfast*

1 cup of high-fiber cereal (such as Fiber One or All-Bran)

1 cup of almond milk

1 cup of orange juice

*Snack*

*Tropical Delight* smoothie, page 104

*Lunch*

1 large chicken breast, grilled or broiled
Pasta salad made with 1 cup of cooked whole wheat or gluten-free pasta,
     1 tablespoon of chopped onion, 2 tablespoons of chopped red pepper,
     Italian seasonings to taste, and 1 teaspoon of olive oil
1 sliced of fresh tomato

*Snack*

Handful of almonds

*Dinner*

5 ounces of tilapia, broiled
1 cup of brown rice
1 cup of steamed asparagus
1 tossed mixed green salad drizzled with 2 tablespoons of light salad dressing

*Total Calories: 1,791*

## Day 7 (Maintenance Cheat Day)

*Breakfast*

1 whole-grain bagel topped with 1 tablespoon of peanut butter or almond butter
1 cup of low-fat cottage cheese
1 medium peach

*Snack*

1 medium banana

*Lunch*

Turkey sandwich: 2 slices of multigrain, gluten-free bread with 3 slices of fat-free turkey ham, 1 slice of Swiss cheese, 2 lettuce leaves, 2 slices of tomato, and 1 tablespoon of dark mustard or mashed avocado

*Snack*

1 medium pear

*Dinner*

2 slices (⅙ to ⅛ of the pie) of pepperoni pizza
1 tossed salad with 2 tablespoons of light dressing
1 light beer (12 ounces)

*Total Calories: 2,063*

# 7-DAY MEAL PLAN: 2,000 CALORIES

## Day 1

*Breakfast*

2 whole-grain waffles with 2 tablespoons of sugar-free maple syrup
2 slices of turkey bacon
1 cup of orange juice

*Snack*

*A+ Smoothie*, page 105

*Lunch*

Chicken Caesar salad at a restaurant
1 bread stick

---

**Restaurant Calorie Red Alert!**

Chicken Caesar salads are often loaded with calories, ranging from 300 to 600 calories per serving. To manage those calories, order the dressing on the side and ask that it be prepared without croutons.

---

*Snack*

1 cup of sliced strawberries
1 cup of low-fat yogurt (your favorite flavor)

*Dinner*

1 sirloin steak, grilled or broiled
*Dolvett's Mock Mashed Potatoes*, page 123, with 1 teaspoon of trans-fat-free
    margarine
1 tossed green salad with 2 tablespoons of fat-free dressing
1 whole-grain dinner roll

---

*Total Calories: 1,978*

## Day 2

*Breakfast*

2 slices of *Biggest Winner French Toast*, page 108, 1 tablespoon of sugar-free
 maple syrup or honey
1 cup of fresh blueberries
1 cup of coconut milk

*Snack*

1 protein bar (with at least 20 grams of protein)

*Lunch*

Peanut butter and jelly sandwich: 2 slices of multigrain, gluten-free bread spread
 with 2 tablespoons of peanut butter and 1 tablespoon of all-fruit spread or
 sugar-free jelly
1 medium apple

*Snack*

Handful of almonds or walnuts
2 fresh apricots or 1 medium peach

*Dinner*

6 ounces of baked or broiled tilapia or other white fish
Pasta salad made with 1 cup of cooked whole wheat or gluten-free pasta,
 1 tablespoon of chopped onion, 2 tablespoons of chopped red pepper,
 Italian seasonings to taste, and 1 teaspoon of olive oil
1 cup of steamed mixed vegetables
1 mixed green salad drizzled with 1 teaspoon of olive oil and 2 tablespoons of
 balsamic vinegar

*Total Calories: 1,896*

## Day 3

*Breakfast*

2 to 3 ounces of smoked salmon

1 medium whole-grain bagel, spread with 1 tablespoon of reduced-fat
  cream cheese

1 cup of orange juice

*Snack*

1 cup of low-fat yogurt (your favorite flavor)

1 cup of fresh strawberries

*Lunch*

2 (3-ounce) grilled or broiled lean ground turkey patties

1 tablespoon of reduced-sugar ketchup, or 1 tablespoon of mustard

1 cup of brown rice

1 tomato, sliced

½ green bell pepper, sliced

*Snack*

Handful of almonds or walnuts

*Dinner*

10 boiled shrimp served over 1 cup of whole wheat or gluten-free angel hair pasta
  and sprinkled with 2 tablespoons of Parmesan cheese, tossed with 1 tablespoon
  of olive oil

1 cup of Italian green beans

*Total Calories: 1,953*

## Day 4 (Maintenance Cheat Day)

*Breakfast*

Egg and muffin: 1 whole wheat toasted English muffin with 1 fully cooked egg,
   1 slice of cheddar cheese, and 2 strips of turkey bacon
1 cup of orange juice

*Snack*

A+ *Smoothie*, page 105

*Lunch*

½ Reuben sandwich at a deli (split it with a friend!)

### Restaurant Calorie Red Alert!

Did you know that the average calorie count in a
Reuben sandwich is 770? That's why I recommend
splitting deli sandwiches. If you make one at
home, use reduced-fat Swiss cheese and fat-free
dressing.

*Snack*

1 cup of low-fat yogurt (your favorite flavor)

*Dinner*

*Oriental Chicken with Hot Garlic Sauce*, page 116
1 cup of brown rice
2 glasses (5 ounces each) of white wine

*Total Calories: 2,257*

## Day 5

*Breakfast*

*Italian Frittata*, page 107
2 slices of multigrain, gluten-free toast with 2 teaspoons of trans-fat-free
    margarine
1 medium banana

*Snack*

*Rise and Grind Smoothie*, page 104

*Lunch*

Turkey sandwich: 2 slices of multigrain, gluten-free bread with 3 slices of fat-free
    turkey ham, 1 slice of Swiss cheese, 2 lettuce leaves, 2 slices of tomato, and
    1 tablespoon of dark mustard or mashed avocado

*Snack*

1 protein bar (with at least 20 grams protein)
1 cup of almond milk

*Dinner*

5 ounces of baked turkey breast
1 medium sweet potato
1 cup of steamed asparagus
1 Skinny Cow ice cream sandwich

*Total Calories: 1,925*

## Day 6

*Breakfast*

4 scrambled egg whites
2 slices of cinnamon and raisin toast
½ cantaloupe

*Snack*

*Rise and Grind Smoothie*, page 104

*Lunch*

Roast beef and Swiss sandwich: 3 slices of roast beef, 1 slice of Swiss cheese,
    2 slices of onion, 2 slices of tomato, 1 tablespoon of Russian salad dressing,
    served on 2 slices of rye bread
1 medium apple

*Snack*

5 whole wheat crackers with 2 tablespoons of peanut butter
1 cup of reduced-sodium vegetable juice

*Dinner*

2 large baked chicken thighs
*Maple Orange Mashed Sweet Potatoes*, page 122
1 cup of steamed asparagus with 1 teaspoon of trans-fat-free margarine
1 cup of pineapple chunks, fresh or canned in juice

*Total Calories: 1,975*

## Day 7 (Maintenance Cheat Day)

*Breakfast*

½ cup of fat-free granola
1 cup of coconut milk
1 medium banana

*Snack*

1 medium apple

*Lunch*

2 beef tacos, made with soft low-carb flour tortillas
1 serving (½ cup) of black beans
1 cup of sliced fresh strawberries

*Snack*

*Tropical Delight* smoothie, page 104

*Dinner*

*Dinner at an Italian restaurant*:
1½ cups of fettuccine Alfredo
1 tossed green salad with 1 tablespoon of Italian dressing
1 glass (5 ounces) of white zinfandel wine or any type of white wine

*Total Calories: 2,190*

---

### Restaurant Calorie Red Alert!

My program is all about allowing you to enjoy your favorite foods now and then. If one of your favorites is fettuccine Alfredo, know that restaurant entrées of this amazing dish contain between 600 and 1,200 calories. My advice: Just eat half and save the rest for another meal.

---

# 7-DAY MEAL PLAN: 2,300 CALORIES

## Day 1

### Breakfast

1 cup of low-fat cottage cheese
1 cup of fruit cocktail, canned in juice
2 slices of multigrain, gluten-free bread, spread with all-fruit jam or sugar-free jelly

### Snack

1 medium banana

### Lunch

Roast beef and Swiss sandwich: 3 slices of roast beef, 1 slice of Swiss cheese, 2 slices of onion, 2 slices of tomato, 1 tablespoon of Russian salad dressing, served on 2 slices of rye bread
1 medium apple

### Snack

*A+ Smoothie*, page 105

*Dinner*

5 ounces of chicken breast, grilled or broiled

1 cup of brown rice

1 tossed green salad with salad veggies such as chopped tomato and onion, drizzled with 2 tablespoons of light salad dressing

1 cup of low-fat yogurt (your favorite flavor)

*Total Calories: 2,286*

## Day 2

*Breakfast*

4 scrambled egg whites

1 cup of oatmeal with 1 tablespoon of honey and ½ cup of almond milk

1 cup of pineapple chunks, fresh or canned in juice

*Snack*

*A+ Smoothie*, page 105

*Lunch*

1 grilled chicken sandwich on a whole-grain bun topped with lettuce and tomato and 1 tablespoon of light mayonnaise

1 cup of *Veggistrone*, page 124

1 medium orange

*Snack*

Protein bar (with at least 20 grams of protein)

### Dinner

5 ounces of broiled or grilled salmon

1 medium sweet potato with 1 tablespoon of sugar-free maple syrup

1 cup of steamed asparagus with 1 teaspoon of trans-fat-free margarine

1 tossed green salad with 2 tablespoons of light salad dressing

1 cup of vanilla frozen yogurt

*Total Calories: 2,284*

## Day 3

### Breakfast

1 medium whole-grain bagel, spread with 1 tablespoon of reduced-fat cream cheese

1 medium apple

1 cup of almond milk

### Snack

5 whole wheat crackers

2 ounces of cheddar cheese

1 medium orange

### Lunch

2 (3-ounce) grilled or broiled lean ground turkey or chicken patties

1 sliced tomato

Pasta salad made with 1 cup of cooked whole wheat or gluten-free pasta, 1 tablespoon of chopped onion, 2 tablespoons of chopped red pepper, Italian seasonings to taste, and 1 teaspoon of olive oil

*Snack*

Protein bar (with at least 20 grams of protein)

*Dinner*

5 ounces of grilled or broiled lean sirloin steak
*Sweet Potato Fries*, page 123
1 cup of steamed mixed vegetables
1 tossed green salad, drizzled with 1 tablespoon of light salad dressing

*Total Calories: 2,268*

## Day 4 (Maintenance Cheat Day)

*Breakfast*

1 cup of cooked oatmeal with 1 tablespoon of honey
2 hard-boiled eggs
1 cup of sliced strawberries

*Snack*

*Peachy Keen Shake*, page 106

*Lunch*

2 slices (⅙ to ⅛ of the pie) of pepperoni pizza
1 tossed green salad, drizzled with 2 tablespoons of light salad dressing

*Snack*

15 to 20 fat-free flour tortilla snack chips dipped in ½ cup of salsa

*Dinner*

*Dinner at a steak house:*
8-ounce prime rib
1 serving garlic mashed potatoes
1 Caesar side salad

*Total Calories: 2,794*

## Restaurant Calorie Red Alert!

Steak house dinners can really rack up the calories. Take the dinner above, for example: the prime rib is 420 calories; the garlic mashed potatoes, 305; and the Caesar side salad, 330. Do the math: 1,055 calories for one meal. I know I keep harping on it, but you need to develop an almost encyclopedic knowledge of the calories in your favorite restaurant foods if you want to keep your weight off!

## Day 5

*Breakfast*

1 cup of shredded wheat
1 cup of almond milk
2 slices of Canadian bacon
1 medium banana, sliced

*Snack*

*Tropical Delight* smoothie, page 104
Handful of almonds

*Lunch*

1 cup of tomato soup (made with water)

1 grilled ham and cheese sandwich: 2 slices of multigrain, gluten-free bread, 1 slice
of cheddar cheese, 1 slice of fat-free ham, and 2 teaspoons of trans-fat-free
margarine, grilled on the stovetop

1 cup of pineapple chunks, fresh or canned in juice

*Snack*

5 whole wheat crackers spread with 1 tablespoon of peanut butter or almond
butter

1 cup of reduced-sodium vegetable juice

*Dinner*

2 medium lamb chops, grilled or broiled

1 cup of cooked couscous

1 cup of steamed green beans

*Total Calories: 2,305*

## Day 6

*Breakfast*

*Italian Frittata*, page 107

1 medium banana

*Snack*

*A+ Smoothie*, page 105

*Lunch*

1 large grilled chicken breast
Pasta salad made with 1 cup of cooked whole wheat or gluten-free pasta,
    1 tablespoon of chopped onion, 2 tablespoons of chopped red pepper,
    Italian seasonings to taste, and 1 teaspoon of olive oil
1 medium apple

*Snack*

Handful of almonds or walnuts

*Dinner*

1 large pork chop, grilled or broiled
1 cup of steamed broccoli topped with 1 teaspoon of trans-fat-free margarine
*Maple Orange Mashed Sweet Potatoes*, page 122
1 cup of unsweetened applesauce
1 cup of low-fat yogurt (your favorite flavor)

*Total Calories: 2,351*

## Day 7 (Maintenance Cheat Day)

*Breakfast*

3 pancakes (any type, 6" diameter) with 1 tablespoon of sugar-free maple syrup
2 slices of Canadian bacon
1 cup of sliced strawberries

*Snack*

*Rise and Grind Smoothie*, page 104

*Lunch*

*Fast-food lunch:*
Cheeseburger with bun, lettuce, and tomato
Medium order of regular fries

---

### Restaurant Calorie Red Alert!

Now, about those fries: A large order contains 500 calories; a medium order, 380 calories; and a small order, 230 calories. Those calories really rack up! If you've just gotta have a taste of fries, order the kiddie portion. It's only about 100 calories.

---

*Dinner*

½ barbecued chicken
1 cup of creamy coleslaw
½ cup of baked beans
1 slice of pecan pie
1 light beer

---

*Total Calories: 2,707*

As a parting shot to this chapter: If you mess up your plan, rebound immediately—at your very next meal. Do not, I repeat, do not beat yourself up over a slip. Slips will happen. The key to long-term maintenance is not letting a binge turn into a week of binge eating.

I'm not saying it will be a cakewalk. It won't. But the job of a living healthy, fit life falls on nobody else's shoulders but yours. And you can do it!

# 9 The 3-1-2-1 Lifestyle

I may be a personal trainer and I may appear on *The Biggest Loser*, but let me tell you who the real experts are: people who have lost weight, gotten in shape, and stayed that way permanently. They're the ones who have discovered the real secrets of health and fitness. Over the years, I've talked to former clients and successful "losers" to find out their best, most effective strategies for staying lean and healthy for a lifetime. In this chapter, I'll share with you what I've learned.

## STAY IN MOTION

Just about everyone I've known who has been successful at keeping their weight off has kept up with their workouts—at least 4 times a week, sometimes more. You'll definitely have an easy time maintaining your ideal weight if you stay active. That doesn't mean doing the same old routine every day, either. Change things up. Don't ever get comfortable in your workouts. Do different styles of workouts in order to use different muscle groups. When you mix it up with new activities, you're shaping and sculpting overlooked muscles. Your body will continue to lean out in different areas, and you'll maintain muscle and tone other areas.

Some specifics: If you're accustomed to doing a cycling class, get a mountain bike and go biking outside on different types of terrains. Play sports. Or do some gardening (digging and weeding incinerate calories). Fulfill your dream running a marathon or a triathlon. At night, hit the nightspots and shake your tail feathers for a workout. There are plenty of ways to stay active—without ever getting bored.

At one time or another, we've all read that putting more activity into our day is a simple way to burn more calories. Well, it's true. For example, let's say you vacuum your house 3 times a week, for an hour each time. You use up 480 calories a week. That might not seem like much, except in a year you've expended 24,960 calories, or 7 pounds. Did you know that making photocopies burns up to 215 calories an hour? If you did that twice a week for a year, you'd burn off about 6 pounds. Lifestyle activities burn up a lot of calories, which means you can drop pounds almost automatically as long as you move around more.

So do a lot of lifestyle activities. Some examples: Climb the stairs instead of riding elevators and escalators. Do some calf raises anytime you're waiting in line; this means simply rising up and down on your toes while standing in place. On errands, park your

| Lifestyle Activity | Length of Time | Calories Burned per Week | Pounds Lost in 1 Year |
|---|---|---|---|
| Take the stairs instead of the elevator or escalator. | 10 minutes, 5 times a week | 1,225 calories | 18 pounds |
| Play actively with your children. | 3 hours, 3 times a week | 780 calories | 12 pounds |
| Wash your own car, instead of taking it to the car wash. | 1 hour, once a week | 376 calories | 6 pounds |
| Take an exercise break at work or home. Get up, walk around, or pump some resistance bands. | 10 minutes, 15 times a week or 3 times each workday | 600 calories | 9 pounds |
| Walk down the office hallway to deliver a message to colleagues rather than e-mailing them. | 10 minutes, 5 times a week | 200 calories | 3 pounds |
| Go dancing. | 2 hours, once a week | 580 calories | 9 pounds |
| Dig and weed in your garden. | 4 hours a week | 800 calories | 12 pounds |
| Use your cell phone and move around while you talk. | 5 hours a week | 565 calories | 8 pounds |

car far away from your destination to slip in some walking. Do some forward lunges as you run the vacuum or sweeper around your house. Walk briskly through the mall. Perform some biceps curls with your shopping bags. Whatever gets your breathing going or makes you sweat, that's exercise. The chart on page 226 illustrates how to sneak more calorie burning into your life.

Above all, look for the fun factor in exercise. Remember when you were a kid? Weren't you active all the time, climbing trees, playing ball, swimming, and all that? And wasn't it fun? Bring back the kid in you by finding fun activities—like riding your bike, doing some snow sports, or joining a bowling or racquetball league. Whatever relieves the exercise blahs, do it!

Finally, don't neglect strength training as part of your maintenance exercise commitment. It will be enormously effective in helping you manage your weight because added muscle keeps your metabolism charged up for continual fat and calorie burning.

# SELF-MONITORING: KEEP TABS ON YOUR BODY

The successful maintainers I've met and worked with keep themselves in check. I realize you can't have a nutritionist or a trainer at your side 24/7, so you've got to be your own motivator. The best way to do this is through self-monitoring, which essentially means regular weighing, doing a "clothes check," keeping a food journal, and tuning in to your energy levels.

## Regular Weighing

I do support frequent weighing, although the scale can sometimes be so deceiving due to water retention or muscle gain. And a lot of experts caution against it because in certain people, bad news on the scale can cause depression, anxiety, stress, and an unhealthy preoccupation with weight. Nonetheless, weighing can be helpful in maintenance. So make scale hopping one of your new favorite sports! Don't obsess over weighing yourself, but jump on the scale at least every couple of days to see whether your weight is going up or down or stabilizing while on maintenance. If it's going up, then ask yourself why:

Am I overeating?

Did I stop counting calories?

Are my portions too big?

Am I eating too much junk food or having more cheat days than allowed?

Am I skipping exercise sessions?

Did my weight gain happen suddenly or has it been a slow trend?

Could health, pregnancy, or medications be contributing to my weight gain?

Collect this information, and analyze it. Think about what might be going on that led to your weight regain. Are there relevant changes? Are you under stress? Have your eating habits gotten lax? Then problem solve by cleaning up your diet, cutting back on your cheats, increasing your exercise, checking with your doctor, or all of the above, until your weight goes back down.

What I recommend, too, is to give yourself an absolute weight ceiling: a number on the scale you will absolutely not exceed. The majority of successful losers never let themselves gain more than several pounds. For one of my female clients, her weight ceiling is 125 pounds. If she finds herself moving past that number, then she returns to consecutive days of straight clean eating (no cheats) until she gets back under 125 pounds. Knowing your absolute keeps you at your ideal weight; trust me on this one! Watch the scale.

I'd like you to do the following exercise: Write a mission statement about your weight ceiling. Here's an example of what I'm talking about:

My new weight is ___, and I will not exceed ___. I will stay under this ceiling for the next 6 months because I need to practice keeping my weight off. I will stay under my ceiling by staying aware of what I eat, exercising several times a week, eating three meals and two snacks daily, planning my meals, choosing Smart Proteins, Smart Fibers, and Smart Carbs, and checking the calorie count of foods, if I'm not sure of them. Should I exceed my ceiling, I will analyze what I might be doing wrong, and I will correct it. I will make a deliberate effort to return to my goal weight, because it is much easier to lose a few pounds than let my weight creep up so much that it becomes difficult to control. I have been successful on this plan, so I know I can stay successful.

Post your mission statement where you can see it: on your refrigerator, on your mirror, or at your desk at work. Reread it often. Trust me, it will help you stay on track!

## Clothes Check

Watch how your clothes fit too. I'm going to trust that you've bought yourself a store-full of "skinny" clothes that fit you beautifully at your new weight. Fantastic! But if they ever start feeling snug, or you can't move your arms and need help getting out of your shirts, or your profile takes up more space in an airplane seat, get back on the plan. And by the way, if you kept any fat clothes, toss them out or donate them. Leave no clothes that fit you at your previous, higher weight in your closet. Too bad if you have nothing to wear out of the house if you start regaining weight. There's no going back now.

## Food Journaling

Another key part of monitoring is to keep a journal or a record of what you eat each day. I realize that after you've met your goal, you think you've got the whole weight thing conquered. But that's a false sense of security, folks. Don't ease up or get lax. You've now got to master weight maintenance. If you start gaining weight again—and you haven't kept a record what you're eating and the calories in your meals—it's tough to zero in on where you're messing up.

That's why successful maintainers know they must keep tabs on what they eat and the calories of the food eaten. If you find your weight creeping up, start writing down everything you eat so you can see where the surplus calories are coming from. Lots of books and websites give the calorie content of foods. Let's be honest with each other: Overeating is often linked to stress, boredom, depression, and other emotions. One way to break that pattern is to write down what you eat—and why. What situations and emotions were connected to your overeating episode? For instance, if you always reach for a bag of chips after a stressful day at work, find nonfood ways to decompress, such as going for a run, reading a book, or meditating.

## *Check Your Energy Levels*

If you're dragging more than you're doing, your program is off and could lead to weight regain. You may not realize it, but our bodies are programmed for an energy drop between 3 p.m. and 5 p.m. But there are strategies to prevent this so you can stay productive and energized. For starters, check your diet. For lunch, make sure you have plenty of lean proteins, greens, and other low-calorie vegetables. Carbs tend to make us feel sluggish, especially processed carbs. Drink plenty of water too. It has an energizing effect on the body. If your urine is dark colored, rather than pale yellow, that may mean you are not drinking enough. Whatever you do, don't think that another cup of coffee or a candy bar from the vending machine will pick you up. It won't. In fact, it will make you droop.

Stress is an energy vampire, sucking away your stamina. The best remedy is exercise. It increases feel-good endorphins in your body, which will lift anxiety and depression. It stimulates your heart and gets energy-giving oxygen flowing through your blood. These physiological responses directly increase your energy level. Whenever something goes wrong in my life, I head to the gym, run, go to an exercise class, or hop on the treadmill. I love working out. It's a release for me, and I workout anywhere between 5 and 6 days a week. Exercise is my salvation against stress.

Reenergize yourself with quality sleep. If you're having trouble sleeping, you'll be dragging your butt the next day. Plus, sleep deprivation can make you gain weight because it throws certain hormones off-kilter. Good sleep is restorative. It's the time when your body repairs itself. If poor sleep is de-energizing you, you've got to make changes in your routine. Cut back on caffeine drinks and alcoholic beverages. Wind down with a hot bath or good book. But don't look at your computer or smart phone just prior to bedtime. These devices adversely stimulate your mind and make it difficult to get quality shut-eye.

# BUILD A TEAM OF SUPPORT

Support from people is everything when you're losing weight and maintaining your weight loss. We simply perform better when we have a team of loved ones who are rooting for us. At the same time, it's extremely challenging to manage your weight when everyone around you is eating Rocky Road ice cream. One of my team members from season 14 was Lisa. Here was a young lady who stayed with me on the phone and via e-mail every single day after she left the ranch because she was so motivated to become the at-home *Biggest Loser* winner. She had shed 108 pounds while at the ranch. Little did I know that her entire family was following the plan because of the supportive atmosphere she had created at home. Her husband lost 75 pounds, her mom lost 45 pounds, and her kids even slimmed down. Lisa ignited a fire inside her entire family and created a whole new appreciation for healthy living.

You've got to have a good support system to be successful. I'm talking about folks who really care about your goals and your health—no naysayers, no negative people, no critical friends. You don't need that; you need people who can prop you up when you feel like throwing in the towel and ditching your good diet. Communicate with your family and loved ones that you want to keep your weight off and live healthy for good. Hold a family meeting and ask for support. "Please don't ask me to cook a lot of fattening food," you can say. "Let's all eat healthy." At the same time, you'll be modeling good food choices to your kids. More important than what you say to your kids is what you

---

## AFFIRM TO GET FIRM: APPS AND OTHER HIGH-TECH FITNESS TOOLS

These days, the fitness biz has more gadgets than 007. There are a lot of nifty high-tech tools and programs you can use to track your progress and stay motivated—so why not jump on this bandwagon?

If you're like me, I'm always toting around my smartpad and phone. Both represent the latest and greatest ways to establish fitness and health benchmarks and keep track of my progress. Right there in my hand is a way to monitor weight, analyze my jogs or bike rides, and even monitor my heart rate and blood pressure. All you have to do, generally, is download your preferred apps.

I love this trend. If you haven't taken advantage of this technology, do so! I've recommend these tools to clients for several years now. Once they got up to speed with the technology, they realized how little they were actually pushing themselves—and that awareness took them to new levels of intensity and much better results.

These are cool tools that deliver greater fitness, better health, and sustained motivation.

do. When I was a kid, my mom would always buy fruits over packaged treats. That made an impression on me. I thought, "I'm going to do that too."

What should you do if someone isn't supportive? Do your best to tune them out. You've heard the old saying, "The best revenge is living well"? Okay, then: Take the attitude that you'll show them how well you can do on this program. When you get to your goal weight and ideal body shape, just start struttin', and you'll show with your accomplishment just how wrong they were.

## YOU'RE NUMBER ONE

Make yourself priority number one. I bet you're busy taking care of your family, and I bet that leaves little time for yourself. You could be tempted to ditch your program or

### WE DID IT ON DOLVETT'S PROGRAM!

We are a husband and wife who had gotten heavy over the years—to the tune of about 40 pounds each. Looking back, we attribute our problem to eating too many refined carbs for breakfast, lunch, dinner, and snacks. We needed to do something, because life just wasn't fun anymore, and our marriage needed some spark.

Desperate to drop pounds, we had tried just about every diet in the world. We'd always lose weight, but then we'd revert to our old bad habits and gain all the weight back. We had always associated diets with denying ourselves certain foods, and so we really hated dieting. Although we felt very discouraged, we decided to try the 3-1-2-1 Diet. It taught us what to eat and in what portions—with the main meals being a combination of protein and certain types of carbs. It made sense to us.

On other diets, we were always hungry and always craving foods we couldn't have. But the 3-1-2-1 Diet changed all that. We learned to eat foods that were once off-limits, and in the right amounts. Initially, we were afraid of the cheat days. We worried that we'd go overboard, eat too much, and gain weight. But the diet teaches you how to eat your favorite foods without bingeing, so we never felt deprived and we were still losing weight. Once we started eating 5 times a day, hunger became a thing of the past. The pounds started to peel off, and we were thrilled.

We started buying more whole grains and tried to avoid refined flour and sugar, and we changed our snack habits to string cheese, fresh fruit, and almonds. Our meals were healthier versions of the meals we used to eat. We were delighted that we could succeed by having some food every few hours. Snacking on healthy choices tided us over between meals and kept us energized.

We were excited that we started fitting into smaller sizes almost right away. A big part of this was the workout. It really changed our physical conditioning and helped us drop pounds faster. We took Dolvett's advice to make a smoothie and drink it after working out. We do feel that this helped us build just the right amount of muscle. We both lost the 40 pounds and have stayed at our goal weight for almost 2 years now. (Amanda adds that she feels very sexy in her bikini!)

Before with dieting, losing weight was all or nothing. We'd either be on a diet or we'd be overeating like crazy. The 3-1-2-1 Diet gave us balance, and we know that balance is key.

Our tips:

- Lose weight as a couple. This makes dieting so much easier. When you eat the same foods as your partner, you keep each other accountable. Working out together can strengthen a relationship too. (If your spouse or partner doesn't need to lose weight, he or she can still benefit from healthier food choices.)
- Go grocery shopping with a list of healthy foods, and stick to that list. We like to go to the store together; it's just one more level of accountability.
- Be proud of your new body and buy great clothes to show it off. (We threw away our fat clothes.)

*—Amanda and Richard B.*

be sporadic with it. Don't! Think of it this way: If you take care of yourself, you'll be better able to take care of those you love. I'm giving you the same advice you hear on airplanes all the time: Put your oxygen mask on first, then your child's. There are times in your life when you come first. When you do that, your kids and family are the beneficiaries.

And, as with diet, it's important for your family to see Mom or Dad engaged in activities and healthy exercise habits. Parents whose kids see them putting on exercise clothes and heading to the gym for a workout or a fitness class, yoga, or Zumba, are sending a powerful message: "These are the things I do to stay healthy, and you should too."

Parents or not, many of the successful losers I've met have developed a healthy sort of selfishness: They prioritize the things they enjoy, such as getting a massage or having a makeover, for example. Those kinds of activities give you moments to celebrate and appreciate all your hard work—and see it pay off.

## REMEMBER WHY YOU LOST THE WEIGHT

One of the toughest parts of maintenance is staying at your goal weight. That's why I love hearing from successful losers about how they stay the course. One person I know keeps old photos of her former fat self around to remind her of what life was like when she was overweight.

I'd love for you to take a moment and reflect on why you lost the weight:

Jot down your top five reasons for not wanting to regain your weight. Maybe it's because you love your new thin, fit appearance. Maybe you don't want to huff and puff anymore going up stairs. Or maybe it is for health reasons, like preventing diabetes or heart disease. Whatever motivates you, write it down here.

1. _____

2. _____

3. _____

4. _____

5. _____

Some of my clients wrote things like: *I look fitter now. I feel more energetic. I love shopping for clothes now. I'm not self-conscious about my size anymore.*

Next, write down the five best habits you learned that will keep your weight off. Some examples are portion control, being aware of calories, food choices, learning how to cheat appropriately, or making workouts fun.

1. _____

2. _____

3. _____

4. _____

5. _____

Here are some entries I've read from my clients: *I plan my meals and take my lunch to work with me. I choose low-fat varieties of foods. I concentrate on eating more vegetables and fruits. I don't eat second helpings. I schedule my workouts into my week. I remind myself about how great I feel after going to the gym. I exercise harder on my cheat days to compensate for the extra calories. I weigh and measure my food to make sure my portion sizes are correct. I eat more slowly.*

There is so much to be gained by losing weight. True, the positive change in your appearance is huge. But there's also the improvement in how you feel about yourself—the general feeling of well-being and greater self-esteem. And how about the reversal in the bad side effects of being overweight? Perhaps your blood pressure has dropped or you're off blood-pressure meds. Maybe your bad cholesterol is history. Or maybe your blood sugar is under control. And certainly, the risk of developing these problems is a thing of the past.

I see these positive health changes in people every season on *The Biggest Loser.* In fact, a team of scientists documented them in a research study and reported their findings in the *American Journal of Medicine* in 2011. This information is such powerful stuff that I have to share it with you.

The study looked into the effects of weight loss, exercise, and calorie restriction on serious health issues such as blood-sugar control, cholesterol and triglycerides, inflammation, and artery health in seventeen *Biggest Loser* contestants over the course of seven months. These issues are all markers of heart health and risk factors for deadly cardiovascular disease.

As usually happens on the show, the contestants lost a lot of weight and body fat—an average of 39 percent of their weight and 66 percent of their body fat. They did it by changing some very bad habits. Consider that before appearing on the show, a lot of contestants were consuming 7,000 to 10,000 calories a day. Then they drop down to 1,200 to 1,800 calories a day, and the weight drops too.

The upshot of these results was a dramatic improvement in all the markers I mentioned above. The contestants' insulin and blood sugar were under control; their arteries got more flexible and therefore able to pump blood more normally; and their blood fats (cholesterol and triglycerides) improved. Not to get too technical, but the researchers observed increases in a protein hormone called adiponectin. This chemical is secreted by your fat cells. It helps the body burn fat and use insulin normally (so that glucose can enter cells for energy), and prevents cells on the interior lining of arteries from getting inflamed (and eventually causing the arteries to clog). When levels of adiponectin go up, your risk of heart disease falls. So just think: By losing weight, you're probably adding a lot of healthy years to your life.

## YOUR CHECKLIST FOR MAINTENANCE

I'll be honest with you. We all face barriers when it comes to weight maintenance. On the next chart, identify your barriers. Answer yes or no, and be honest with yourself. If something pops up as a barrier, then list some possible solutions and follow through.

I'll admit that maintenance is the greatest challenge on your weight-loss journey, because we have so many temptations and more access to bad choices over good ones. Don't let the bad choices con you. Fortify yourself against them by dialing in to what you do and what you choose: preparing healthy, fat-burning meals...packing healthier lunches and snacks...moving more...feeling better...regaining self-control...not giving up even when occasionally giving in...and most of all, regaining hope that staying at your ideal weight is possible.

|  | Yes | No | Sometimes | Solutions |
|---|---|---|---|---|
| Do you work out at least 4 times a week? | | | | |
| Do you vary your routine? | | | | |
| Do you make your workouts fun? | | | | |
| Do you include strength training in your weekly workouts? | | | | |
| Do you build activity into your daily routine? | | | | |
| Do you weigh yourself regularly? | | | | |
| Do you have an absolute weight ceiling you will not exceed? | | | | |
| Do your clothes fit your new size? | | | | |
| Do you write down everything you eat? | | | | |
| Do you carefully watch your portions? | | | | |
| Are your calories carefully calculated? | | | | |
| Do you eat regular meals and snacks throughout the day? | | | | |
| Are you following the 3-1-2-1 plan as closely as possible? | | | | |
| Have there been any recent increases in your weight? If so, what will you do about them? | | | | |

# Part Four

*More Tools from My Toolbox*

# 10 Supplement Power

Nutritional supplements are a tool I believe in and live by. When it comes to supplements, I support a synergistic approach, in which a healthy diet, regular exercise, and supplements are combined as a total program. Supplements and other things can help but the real help comes from a healthy lifestyle. Although you do not have to gulp down handfuls of pills to be successful on this diet and exercise plan, I wanted to write a chapter on supplements, to give you some new information on how they can help your body in various ways, should you choose this extra edge.

When I became certified as a personal trainer many years ago, I spent a lot of time doing research on nutrition and supplements. I studied the programs of people in really great shape, from well-known trainers to athletes. I read the scientific literature on nutritional supplements, and I began to put the information to use to improve myself and to improve my clients' results. The more I worked with people on supplements, the more I realized what worked and what didn't. That's where I think I'm so much different from many fitness authors and trainers. I developed my diet, supplement strategies, and workout program at a grassroots level, learning and observing firsthand what was effective and what was bogus. I'm not going to pass on information to you unless I'm positive it will work for you. That's just the way I roll. What I'll talk about here is a supplement program that has impact based on the results I've seen with my clients for many, many years of personal training.

Supplements have advanced so much from the popular "one-a-day" multivitamins of the past, although taking a multiple is important for filling in possible nutritional gaps in your diet. Now we have very targeted antioxidants, amino acids, supplemental fats, and other nutrients that can do everything from repairing cells to burning fat to increasing muscle tone.

For starters, let me ask you: Before taking any sort of supplement, are you doing everything you can to improve your body through exercise and diet?

If you answered yes, I congratulate you. Now, if you want a bigger nutritional boost, then, by all means, take supplements.

Here are some supplements you may want to consider. I've grouped them into specific categories.

## METABOLIC SUPPORT: MULTIVITAMINS AND MINERALS

No rocket science here, but it's surprising just how many of my clients didn't take a multiple vitamin and mineral supplement. With store shelves filled with all sorts of supplements, it's easy to forget about the basic multivitamin/mineral. But please don't. Supplementing with this one helps metabolism, supports muscle growth, and basically regulates almost every biochemical system in your body. (Food is packed with vitamins and minerals too; see the chart on pages 243–244 for all the nutrients you get from the foods on the 3-1-2-1 Diet). If you take nothing else, take one of these—and do it habitually. Make this part of your daily routine, like brushing your teeth. Keep your bottle of vitamins and minerals next to your toothbrush, in fact, or your coffeemaker as a reminder.

An all-purpose multivitamin/mineral supplement covers all your nutritional bases, plus has a few added health benefits. Even if you follow the most nutritionally sound and clean diet plan, particularly if you work out hard, you could be running low in a few key vitamins and minerals needed to support your progress. That's where a good multi comes in handy.

Read the supplement label and make sure that it gives you at least 100 percent of the daily requirement of most of the vitamins and minerals listed. Take it with a meal because most multivitamins/minerals are absorbed best with food.

### Vitamin D

I'd like to call out one vitamin from the lineup: vitamin D. A lot of us are shockingly low in it. That's because one of the main sources of vitamin D is sunlight, and many of

## FOODS AND MULTIVITAMINS

*Here's a breakdown of select vitamins and minerals in a common multivitamin and good food sources of each nutrient.*

| Vitamin or Mineral | How It Works | Food Sources on the 3-1-2-1 Diet |
|---|---|---|
| Vitamin A | Helps your body repair and build itself | Sweet potatoes, yams, spinach, carrots, cantaloupe, and peppers |
| Vitamin C | Necessary for the formation of collagen, which holds your body together; it also helps the body absorb iron and is important for wound repair | Peppers, oranges, grapefruits, and kiwifruit |
| Vitamin D | Necessary for bone growth and development; may prevent many life-threatening illnesses, including certain forms of cancer | Salmon and tuna; sunlight |
| Vitamin E | Protects muscles from excessive damage and may improve exercise performance | Almonds |
| Vitamin K | Helps manufacture sugar in your muscles (glycogen) for energy; involved in normal blood clotting | Spinach, kale, parsley, and collard and turnip greens |
| B vitamins (thiamin, riboflavin, niacin, B6, folic acid, B12) | Involved in carbohydrate metabolism, growth, muscle tone, energy production, and the health of cells | Eggs, green leafy vegetables, legumes, nuts and seeds, peas, fish, and poultry |
| Biotin | Helps the body break down fat | Nuts, pork, whole grains, and legumes |

*continued*

| Vitamin or Mineral | How It Works | Food Sources on the 3-1-2-1 Diet |
|---|---|---|
| Pantothenic acid | Helps the body burn fat and increase energy | Avocado, broccoli, kale, poultry, whole-grain cereals, and potatoes |
| Calcium | Involved in bone formation, muscle growth, and nerve transmission | Nonfat yogurt, broccoli, fortified almond and coconut milks, and green leafy vegetables |
| Phosphorus | Helps metabolize carbo-hydrates, protein, and fat; involved in growth and repair; stimulates energy production | Nonfat yogurt, salmon, halibut, poultry, and beef |
| Magnesium | Helps metabolize carbo-hydrates and protein; involved in neuromuscular contractions | Green leafy vegetables, bananas, avocados, legumes, nuts, and whole grains |
| Zinc | Helps regulate growth and wound healing; promotes immunity | Oysters, poultry, crab, and red meat |
| Selenium | Protects immunity and protects cells against damage | Tuna, cod, and turkey (breast meat) |
| Chromium | Regulates blood sugar and helps metabolize fat | Broccoli, potatoes |
| Potassium | Helps maintain normal water balance in the body; stimulates nerve impulses from cell to cell; and helps the body convert blood sugar to muscle energy | Bananas, apricots, oranges, broccoli, squash, and nuts |

us go out of our way to avoid spending time in the sun. Stories about skin cancer don't help, either. But too much hiding out means we're missing out on a great nutrient for fat burning.

Mostly known for making bones stronger, vitamin D increases the "thermic effect of food." This phrase refers to the calories burned during the digestion of food. Vitamin D also seems to boost overall fat burning, studies now show. Moreover, Vitamin D is unusual among other vitamins because it acts like a hormone in the body, sending chemical messages back and forth and telling the body to stop storing fat. When levels of vitamin D are low, it's bad news for your shape. A chemical called "circulating parathyroid hormone" starts to rise in response to a lack of vitamin D. This reaction triggers weight gain in the form of body fat.

You can have your vitamin D levels tested when you get your annual blood work done. If you're low in this important nutrient, your doc may have you supplement. Most physicians recommend 1,000 to 2,000 IU of vitamin D3 (a form that is highly usable by the body) 1 to 2 times a day with food. Good food sources of vitamin D are tuna and herring.

## Protein Powder

I love protein powder! It's a must-have, along with your multivitamin/mineral supplement. It's an excellent source of protein, and protein is the number one nutrient for developing attractive, lean-and-mean body contours. Add protein powder to your smoothies for a good jolt of this powerful nutrient.

There are lots of choices when purchasing protein powder, and it can be confusing. There are three types I recommend:

*Whey protein powder.* Whey makes up about one-fourth of the protein in milk. Though I'm not a fan of milk, I love whey. It's among the best proteins you can take. It contains minerals and all the essential amino acids and, due to its unique molecular makeup, is absorbed really well. Microscopically, whey is comprised of peptides, tiny necklaces of amino acids that the body can easily put to use. Some of these peptides help your body burn fat. Whey also helps repair muscle, enhances muscle development, and improves immunity against disease.

*Brown rice protein powder.* As you might suspect, brown rice powder comes from whole-grain brown rice and is a great source of well-absorbed protein. It has a mild flavor and tastes great in all sorts of shakes and smoothies. I consider it a good protein to take before and after workouts. Also, this protein powder is a terrific choice if you're following a plant-based diet.

*Hemp protein powder.* I know what you're thinking: Hemp? Can I get high on that? Sorry, not this kind. This type of hemp contains only traces of THC, a psychoactive substance in marijuana. In fact, there's so little THC in this hemp that even if you ate nothing but hemp foods, you still wouldn't take in enough THC to groove at a rock concert. Hemp protein powder is high in heart-healthy omega-3 fatty acids. It is also easily digested with a direct route to your muscles and contains well-balanced amounts of all essential amino acids.

Each of these protein powders provides specific benefits that work in symbiotic ways with each other to drive fat burning and muscle development. For this reason, I rotate my clients through different protein powders, or have them combine protein powders in their shakes and smoothies, say ½ scoop of whey protein combined with ½ scoop of hemp protein. Try that, and you'll get the best of each protein powder.

## Timing Your Protein Supplement

I admit that I've ripped a few pages from the bodybuilder playbook. Love 'em or hate 'em, bodybuilders know a lot about how to get the most from nutrition, and they've got lower-than-low body-fat levels to prove it. Don't worry; I'm not going to turn you into a bodybuilder—just the best physical version of yourself. However, I am going to give you some insider information that bodybuilders and athletes have known and used for years: how to time your protein supplements for the very best results.

Absolutely the very best time to swill a protein smoothie is after your workout. I don't want to get too technical, but within the first hour after exercising, your muscles are hungry for all the nutrients they can get. They want carbs, they want protein, and they are primed to soak both nutrients up, if they're present. Plus, drinking a protein-and-carb-fortified smoothie (like those made with fruit, nut milk, and protein powder) right after training creates a situation in your body that is conducive to muscle growth and repair. Both the protein and carbs jack up your muscles' ability to rebuild themselves, replenish your glycogen stores, and ease off on the amount of fat that your body stores.

The next most important time is immediately before workouts. Having a shake before training helps you energize your body with fuel. The more fuel available, the harder you can work out. And the harder you work out, the more fat you burn and muscle you create.

The third best time for a protein smoothie: first thing in the morning. Your body needs morning fuel because it has been fasting overnight. The sooner you get some quality protein and carbs in your body, the less chance you risk of your body breaking down muscle for energy. That's why as soon as I get up, I like to blend up a smoothie. I know it will halt that breakdown and start restoring any muscle protein I lost during the night.

## Water Balance

### Dandelion

I've had a lot of women clients who complain of water retention—otherwise known as bloat—and the false weight gain it produces. You can be losing body fat but retaining water, and your hard work won't show up on the scale or in the mirror. What gives? Your body is holding on to water just under your skin. This condition is caused by eating salty or sugary foods, being dehydrated, or undergoing hormonal swings. Honestly, the best remedy is to drink enough water throughout the day, as I have recommended. I know it doesn't make sense, but drinking water flushes out excess water.

Another solution is to consider supplementing with dandelion, a natural herbal diuretic. It's made from the leaves or root of that pesky weed that grows in your lawn every year—the one with the puffball seeds that kids like to blow. Dandelion works by encouraging the kidneys to excrete sodium chloride, while sparing potassium. Taking dandelion could help you drop up to 3 pounds of ugly bloat in just a day.

Check your health food store for products formulated as capsules or tinctures. Herbalists and health practitioners usually recommend taking 1 gram of dandelion root in capsule form twice a day for water retention. Or you can make a tea by dropping some dandelion tincture in a cup of warm water. (If using a tincture, note what the manufacturer recommends as dosages.) Don't take or drink more than is recommended, though. You could lose too much water, and that's unhealthy. You could flush your system of electrolytes, namely sodium and potassium, which enable communication between cells.

In addition to its diuretic properties, dandelion has been shown to be an antioxidant. (Antioxidants help prevent the cell damage that leads to cancer, heart disease, Alzheimer's disease, and other life-threatening conditions.)

## Coconut Water

Here's one of the finest supplement drinks I've found for hydrating during workouts and rehydrating afterward: coconut water. Don't confuse it with coconut milk, which is a blend of the white meat of coconut with water. Coconut water is the stuff that sloshes around inside the coconut fruit. In the Caribbean, you'd punch a hole in the coconut husk, insert a straw, and sip the slightly sweet liquid inside. Stateside, you can buy bottled or canned coconut water right off the supermarket shelf, and it's just as tasty as you'd find in the tropics.

Coconut water has a pretty impressive résumé of benefits. For starters, it's an "isotonic" beverage. That means it has the same level of electrolyte balance we have in our bodies. Electrolytes include potassium, sodium, calcium, and magnesium—minerals often lost in sweat—which is why coconut water makes a terrific natural sports drink to replace those nutrients. Coconut water, in fact, contains more potassium than a banana and 15 times more potassium than typical sports drinks. Unlike sports drinks, it contains no dyes, artificial sweeteners, added sugar, or preservatives. More hydrating than water, coconut water is also rich in vitamin C, which is good for immunity.

Because it's low in fat, sugar, and calories, coconut water is a good dieting tool. It makes a great snack or breakfast beverage. Each 8 ounces contains only 45 calories.

I wouldn't exactly call it a cure-all, but some advocates of coconut water claim it has antiviral and antifungal properties, meaning it may be able to help your body better fight viruses, including colds and bladder infections.

So check out coconut water. It's a healthy choice and fits in perfectly with the 3-1-2-1 Diet and an active lifestyle.

## Fat Metabolism: CLA and Yohimbine

### CLA

CLA, or conjugated linoleic acid, is a healthy fat that has been studied for a long time as a fat burner. It was promoted a decade ago for weight loss, especially if you were a lab rat. Seriously! Since then, though, many more human studies have been done. Now it appears that CLA works for not only lab rats but people too.

One of the most fascinating studies I found was published in the *American Journal of Clinical Nutrition*. The report reviewed CLA studies: The supplement effectively produced fat loss in seven out of the eighteen human studies that were reviewed; eleven other studies showed a more modest fat loss. So the science is looking pretty powerful in support of this supplement. CLA works by blocking the action of a fat-storing enzyme called lipoprotein lipase. When this enzyme is neutralized, your body deposits less fat and burns more fat as fuel.

CLA naturally occurs in the fat component of cow's milk and meat. The operative word here is *fat*. You won't get any CLA from skim milk or nonfat yogurt because it isn't there. Plus, you eat very little of both on my diet, so supplementing with CLA may be a good move.

The recommended dose is typically 3 grams (1 gram at breakfast, another at lunch, and the final dosage at dinner) while dieting and exercising to lose weight. Also, consider taking it after you've reached your goal weight since CLA's benefits increase the longer you use it.

### Yohimbine

The other fat burner I like is yohimbine. Made from the bark of the yohimbe, a tropical African tree, yohimbine is usually marketed as a sexual potency aid for men. In fact, it was the preferred impotence treatment for millions of men around the world before the Viagra craze.

Then various lab tests on yohimbine found that not only did it stimulate, ahem, a man's private part, but it also increased the levels of a stress hormone called norepinephrine in the bloodstream. Norepinephrine stimulates the breakdown of fatty acids in the body, and an increased release of free fatty acids into the blood means you'll burn more stored fat. One recent study I read while writing this book found that when professional soccer players took yohimbine, they lost more body fat, without sacrificing muscle, than those who took a placebo pill.

The usual dosage is to take two 10-milligram doses of yohimbine 2 to 3 times a day with one dose 30 to 60 minutes prior to your workout. This supplement has been studied mostly in men, so I recommend that only men take it.

## Muscle Health: Branched-Chain Amino Acids

Branched-chain amino acids (BCAAs) are used by bodybuilders and exercisers to build muscle, repair muscle, and overcome fatigue. There are three BCAAs: leucine, isoleucine, and valine. They're named BCAAs because if you drew their chemical structure on a piece of paper, your drawing would look like trees with branching limbs. Most BCAA supplements include all three because they need to be taken as a team to work optimally.

What I love about BCAAs is how the body uses them. When you take amino acids (as individual supplements or as a slab of protein-rich meat), they first head to your liver, where they are broken down and used to meet your body's protein requirements. The liver, however, reroutes BCAAs directly to the muscles to be used for building muscle.

The muscles can also use BCAAs, unlike other aminos, directly for energy. This endows BCAAs with two unique characteristics. First, you've heard the term *alternative fuel*, right? Well, BCAAs are like an alternative fuel but for powering your body. In fact, they act almost like carbohydrates. No other aminos behave like this. What happens is that BCAAs convert to glucose (blood sugar), thus providing an alternative energy source to muscle glycogen, which is what your muscles run on normally. In fact, these aminos are so important to energy that if your BCAA stores dip and you're grinding out a lot of cardio, your body will actively break down muscle to get more energy. BCAAs prevent that from happening. Thus, BCAAs may benefit you indirectly by preserving muscle tissue.

Second, during rest, such as after workouts, BCAAs are used for building muscle. This means you definitely want to supplement with them before workouts to drive muscle growth, increase energy, and blunt fatigue, and after your workout to help develop muscle. And because BCAAs drive energy, taking them prior to workouts isn't a bad idea, either.

BCAAs are a supercool pre-workout supplement too. The usual dosage is to take 3 to 5 grams twice daily on an empty stomach, or follow the manufacturer's recommended dosage on the label, since products vary in potency.

## Circulation Support—Arginine

Here we come to one of my favorite supplements: arginine. It's an amino acid whose main job is to form nitric oxide (NO) in the body. (NO is not to be confused with the laughing gas, nitrous oxide, you get while having dental work.) So what's the big deal about NO? It increases blood flow—which means more nutrients and oxygen get delivered to muscles so they can grow, develop, and get more toned. Not surprisingly, arginine has broader benefits to your cardiovascular system as a whole. Research tells us that NO helps prevent fatty acids from building up and sticking to the interior walls of your arteries.

There are other muscle-building benefits of arginine too: It helps the body synthesize protein, and it stimulates the secretion of growth hormone, a substance involved in muscle growth and the breakdown of fat. This is why arginine is so popular with fitness buffs who want greater muscle development and body-fat loss.

Arginine supplements look like they can reduce blood pressure, likely as a result of NO's ability to relax and dilate blood vessels. The ability to strengthen immunity might be another big benefit. White blood cells, which defend the body, use NO to kill bacteria, fungi, and other nasty invaders.

The arginine dosage typically recommended is 2 to 3 grams daily.

## Digestive Health—Chia Seeds

Yes, I'm talking about the plant that sprouts up out of that funky clay pet. The seeds of the chia plant are nutritional dynamos, and I recommend supplementing your diet with them—for a bunch of reasons.

First, these seeds are loaded with antioxidants, protein, omega-3 fats, soluble fiber, vitamins, and minerals. Second, the seeds can help you with weight loss. They soak up 10 to 12 times their weight, forming a satiating gel in your tummy that can curb your desire to overeat. Third, they also slow the digestive process that breaks down carbs and converts them to sugar, which means fewer carbs feeding the fat cells around your midsection.

Chia seeds are native to Mexico and a member of the mint family, though they taste nutty, not minty. *Chia* comes from the Mayan word for strength, which is fitting since Aztec warriors used to eat the seeds for energy prior to going into battle.

How can you tap into all these health benefits? I like sprinkling the seeds into yogurt, cereal, or salads. You can even bake them into foods. All you need are 2 tablespoons a day to get the vitality-boosting benefits of chia seeds.

## General Energy Support—Maca

Maca is a tuber, related to turnips and radishes, and has been grown and eaten by South American locals for approximately 2,000 years. Supposedly, Incan warriors would eat maca prior to battle for stamina. Maca is endowed with vitamins, minerals, protein, carbohydrates, fiber, and fatty acids. Now it's being marketed as a supplement for endurance and strength, with studies supporting its effectiveness. Maca is billed as an "adaptogen." An adaptogen is a substance that helps the body work out harder and prevents excessive damage from the stress of training.

The usual dosage ranges from 200 milligrams to 1 gram a day. Check the manufacturer's recommendations on the label.

# DEVELOP A PERSONAL SUPPLEMENT STRATEGY

No doubt, you're panicking, thinking you need to take every one of these supplements. No, you don't, with the exception, perhaps, of a multivitamin/mineral and a protein powder. But if some of these supplements interest you, then zero in on your choices by figuring out your specific needs.

Ask yourself: Do I need to burn more fat, curb my appetite, tweak my metabolism, get more energy, or work on muscle development?

Then look over the following chart. It provides a snapshot look at how to use these supplements. See where you fit in, and which supplement or supplements might work best. Give your supplements several weeks before deciding whether they are working for you. And don't forget to follow my 3-1-2-1 Diet and exercise plan, and take a multivitamin/mineral daily!

## Supplement Strategies

### You're Overweight and Want Help Burning Off Pounds

| Supplement | How It Works | Usual Dosage |
|---|---|---|
| Whey protein powder | Reputed to be a fat-burner, according to studies | 1 to 3 scoops daily as a part of a smoothie |
| Vitamin D | Increases the thermic effect of food | 1,000 to 2,000 IU of vitamin D3 |
| CLA | Blocks a key fat-storing enzyme | 3 grams daily (1 gram with each main meal); can be used by men and women |
| Yohimbine | Activates a fat-burning hormone | Two 10-milligram doses of yohimbine 2 to 3 times a day with one dose 30 to 60 minutes prior to your workout; recommended for men only |

### You Tend to Overeat and Have Trouble Controlling Your Appetite

| Supplement | How It Works | Usual Dosage |
|---|---|---|
| Protein powder (any type) | Increases satiety (the feeling of fullness in your stomach) | 1 to 3 scoops daily as a part of a smoothie |
| Chia seeds | When taken with fluids, increase in size in the stomach, promoting fullness | 2 tablespoons daily |

### You Want More Energy for Workouts and for Life

| Supplement | How It Works | Usual Dosage |
|---|---|---|
| Protein powder (any type) | Replenishes lost muscle energy and protein after workouts | 1 to 3 scoops daily as a part of a smoothie |
| BCAAs | Serve as an extra fuel source for muscles | 3 to 5 grams twice daily on an empty stomach |

continued

| Maca root | Acts as an adaptogen to provide more energy for more intense workouts | 200 milligrams to 1 gram a day |
|---|---|---|

### You Want to Concentrate on Developing More Muscle

| Supplement | How It Works | Usual Dosage |
|---|---|---|
| Protein powder (any type) | Ensures that your muscles are well supplied for growth and repair | 1 to 3 scoops daily as a part of a smoothie |
| BCAAs | Involved in protein synthesis, plus protect muscle tissue from being broken down for energy | 3 to 5 grams twice daily on an empty stomach |
| Arginine | A factor in increasing oxygen and nutrients to muscles tissue for growth and repair | 2 to 3 grams daily |

### You Are Concerned About Water Retention

| Supplement | How It Works | Usual Dosage |
|---|---|---|
| Dandelion | A natural diuretic that helps the body eliminate excess water | 1 gram of dandelion root in capsule form twice a day for water retention; or drops of an herb tincture in a cup of warm water |
| Coconut water | Helps you stay hydrated, and a properly hydrated body retains less water | 8 ounces after your workout to replenish nutrients lost through sweat, or enjoy it as a hydrating snack |

### You Want to Maintain Your Weight Loss

| Supplement | How It Works | Usual Dosage |
|---|---|---|
| Protein powder (any type) | Helps maintain and repair lean muscle, which in turn helps keep your metabolism healthy | 1 to 3 scoops daily as a part of a smoothie |

| BCAAs | Help maintain lean muscle, which in turn helps keep your metabolism healthy | 3 to 5 grams twice daily on an empty stomach |
|---|---|---|
| CLA | Blocks the action of a fat-storing enzyme, so your body deposits less fat and burns more fat as fuel | 3 grams daily (1 gram with each main meal); can be used by men and women |

# HOW TO PURCHASE QUALITY SUPPLEMENTS

There's a lot of junk out there, so you want to make sure you buy quality supplements. Here's some advice for making a beneficial decision.

Make sure the product is manufactured by a reputable company. An example would be a multivitamin mineral like Centrum, made by Pfizer, a major pharmaceutical company.

Find out if the supplement is supported by solid scientific research. One way to do this is to search PubMed, a huge data bank of clinical studies amassed by the National Library of Medicine. Look for human studies, rather than those performed on lab animals. Other credible sources of supplement information are WebMD (www.webmed .com) and the Mayo Clinic (www.mayoclinic.com). If a claim is made about a supplement, check it out and learn all you can about it from the science.

Read the supplement label to see if it has any sort of "seal of approval." The most credible approvals will come from one of the following: ConsumerLab.com, the Natural Products Association (NPA), or the United States Pharmacopeial Convention (USP).

Is there an expiration date on the supplement label? This is important. There are some supplements, such as calcium and other minerals, that stay potent for several years, while others like vitamins B and C tend to degrade. The Food and Drug Administration doesn't mandate expiration dates on supplements, so many manufacturers don't bother with them. A reputable manufacturer will usually provide one, though.

One more point: Always let your doctor know which supplements you're taking. That said, I hope you can use this information, along with the diet and workout program, to help you get in superb shape and ultimately stay fit, active, and healthy for the rest of your life.

# 11 Real-Life Strategies

At the beginning of this book, I told you that this is a diet for real life. Here's where I want to show you how it works in real-life situations such as socializing, going on vacations, handling special occasions, and unexpected situations that arise when you're just living life. Can you adapt the 3-1-2-1 Diet to all that? You betcha!

One of the things you're finding out about this diet is how truly livable and sustainable it is—through any circumstance or situation that crops up in your life, from a party to travel to times when the going gets tough. Normally, when people go on a diet, things tootle along pretty well, until smack: Life happens. They lose their job. They have to take an unexpected business trip. Someone in the family falls ill. Then all attempts at losing weight and living healthy, no matter how valiant, fall by the wayside.

Thankfully, that unfortunate or unforeseen circumstance usually comes and goes, but the weight gain from falling off the diet wagon is the unwelcome residue of "life happening." If you know what I'm talking about or have experienced it, you know that feelings of failure and utter frustration wash over you, and it's tough to get going again. Big Macs and all-you-can-eat buffets are starting to look good again. You're left wondering, "What does work? I don't want to eat so reactively anymore!" It's not easy to eat clean in certain environments.

Yes, life threw you a curveball, but you're not a failure. It's just that your weight-gaining skills overtook your weight-losing skills. That's where I come in. I want to coach you into reversing that trend by showing you how my 3-1-2-1 Diet automatically strengthens your weight-losing skills and helps you plan for *all* foreseeable possibilities. So let's start the coaching session by talking about something near and dear to my heart: travel.

# TRAVEL STRATEGIES

If you knew how much I travel, you probably wouldn't believe me. One week I might be in New York City meeting with a company; the next week, I might be in Georgia or Virginia visiting family. And somewhere in between, I might be in the Midwest giving a speech to a women's group. I'm on the road so much that even my GPS gets lost.

It would be easy for me to pig out and puff out with all that traveling, yet I don't, because I've trained myself to make better choices under those circumstances. I'm talking about choices so simple that it's hard to believe they could make much of a difference, until you try them yourself and experience their cumulative effect.

Travel—and I'm including vacations in this discussion—presents huge challenges when you're trying to lose weight. You're in unfamiliar surroundings in which food choices are different from what you've stocked in your fridge, and you have less control over how that food is prepared. As a result, you often end up forgetting your program and gaining weight in the process.

No matter what your travel destination, avoid weight gain through good planning. Here's where my 3-1-2-1 Diet really helps: You know you can eat clean on certain days; then you get to "cheat" on 2 days. On your cheat days, allow yourself available treats (but don't binge), then make clean choices on the other days. The latter is easier said than done while traveling or on vacation, however.

Here's what I suggest: Again, always lean toward clean. Whenever possible, choose lean proteins, veggies, salads, fruits, and nuts—whether you're in an airport, on a plane, in a gas station, on a train, in a hotel, at an all-inclusive resort, or on a cruise. If you can pack clean foods, all the better. Think protein bars, almonds, and fruit that won't spoil or bruise easily. If you're at a resort or on a cruise ship, find out if they offer vegetarian, low-carb, and low-fat menus. Whatever you eat, watch your portions—no supersizing! Use Dolvett's Dish to arrange your main meals with Smart Protein, Smart Fiber, and Smart Carbs. Does your alcohol intake increase when you're on vacation? Be honest! If it does, strategize how you will handle this. One strategy you already know about is treating yourself to an alcoholic beverage on your cheat days only. If that doesn't work, then simply figure the calorie counts of your favorite adult beverages into your daily eating plan.

While traveling, stay active. Go to the gym on the cruise ship, or take exercise classes while at sea. Make reservations at a hotel that has a fitness center, and use it. Or pack some resistance bands in your suitcase and work out in your hotel room. Do laps in the pool. Take your running shoes and actually use them!

The other point I must make is this: Focus on other aspects of your trip, rather than the food. Enjoy the people you meet, the locale, the sightseeing, and all the activities.

If you happen to splurge more than you should, don't get bent out of shape. It's not possible to gain huge amounts of weight from one splurge, unless of course the splurge gets stretched out to weeks on end. It's what happens after the splurge that matters. Get back on course right away, whether this means taking a brisk walk or eating one healthy meal. Remembering this will help you bounce back from not-exactly-healthy choices and push you to keep on doing the good stuff. Remember, this is a lifestyle change, not just a diet that lasts as long as your willpower does.

## IT'S YOUR BIRTHDAY AND OTHER SPECIAL OCCASIONS

Watching calories on special occasions like birthdays, weddings, and parties isn't exactly easy. But look at it this way: These occasions give you a great opportunity to practice the concepts I've taught you on the 3-1-2-1 Diet. You can plan your cheat days on those special-occasion days.

Let's say tomorrow is your birthday. I suggest that you eat lightly at lunch and breakfast. Then have your cake and eat it too for your birthday celebration. And that's your cheat day. The key here is planning ahead. Will you have just one piece of birthday cake or two? Which will fit into your cheat-day calorie allotment? Will you have alcohol? Be wise here; alcohol does add calories, and by lowering your inhibitions, it can weaken your resolve to eat within reasonable limits.

Everyone eats and drinks at special occasions, but that doesn't mean you have to stuff yourself. Choosing smaller portions shouldn't be a problem if you set your mind to it. Unwittingly though, family, friends, and partygoers can push food in your face, and lots of it. For these situations, I advise you to prepare yourself with several tactful, polite ways to say "No, thank you." It's easier to deal with these situations if you've planned for them in advance. Practice how to refuse food politely, and don't feel like you need to eat to please other people. These are all choices to be made prior to the event.

And for extra insurance, do some damage control. For example, if you did too much splurging, increase your workout effort the next day. Do a longer workout, or add an extra cardio session to the mix. Push your intensity.

Special occasions are all manageable under my program, and you can still have fun and eat clean without being a party pooper.

## SEASON'S EATINGS: HOLIDAY CELEBRATIONS

Toward the end of the year, the holidays approach. Up until then, you've been cruising along on a nutritious, active path. Then, wham! You're sidetracked by the holidays. One slipup leads to another, then another, and pretty soon, you've got a bottom as big as Frosty's. I don't know about you, but holidays are the time of the year when my bathroom scale starts getting really nervous, because I love to eat.

So here, I want to share some tips to help you make sure that weight doesn't increase as fast as some credit card balances during the holidays:

Work out a few hours before you sit down for a holiday dinner.

Load up on green vegetables at meals; they will always satisfy you.

At the end of your meal, as hard as it might be, opt for fruit instead of a sugary dessert, unless it's your cheat day.

Stay away from casseroles because they are very high in creams and butter and pack lots of calories.

Opt for a lightly sweetened sweet potato, instead of a mashed potato side dish.

Go for the turkey breast; lean turkey is filled with protein.

If you're invited to someone's home, try to politely find out what is being served. If you know your host well, explain that you're watching your diet and volunteer to bring some healthy dishes. Otherwise, decide in advance what you'll eat and plan accordingly.

Fill your plate mostly with salad and veggies, and sample only small portions of high-calorie dishes. You'll control your calories better, without calling attention to your weight-control plans.

At buffets, head for the healthiest foods available. Instead of parking yourself at the buffet table nibbling nonstop, I recommend that you fill your plate and then go sit down somewhere to eat.

If you're the host, you have more control over what it is served. You can plan your holiday meal to include lower-fat and lower-calorie dishes. Depending on the recipes you use, sometimes it's hard to tell the difference between a high-calorie dish and its calorie-downsized counterpart.

Keep a close eye on your portion sizes during the holiday feasts. Enjoy everything that is usually only available during the holidays, but do it in moderation. Indulging in small amounts of holiday treats might not help you lose a lot of weight at this time, but it might help you from raiding the fridge in the middle of the night.

Stay active. Yes, I am harping on this, but unfortunately, it's easy for exercise routines to get derailed during the holidays. But exercise keeps you sane and slim—in three important ways. It relieves stress (who hasn't been stressed-out during holidays?), helps you sleep better, and defrays the caloric cost of candy, pie, gravy and mashed potatoes, and all the other holiday goodies. So regardless of what comes between you and your workout, try not to eliminate it altogether. In fact, I'd recommend that you do more exercising during the holidays!

Focus properly. The holiday season is a time to celebrate good times with family and friends. Try to make the focus more on socializing and less on eating.

Happy holidays, everyone!

## WORKDAY STRATEGIES

Maybe you work in an office where doughnuts, vending machines, and other treats lie around virtually every corner. This is tough and tempting. Your best chance for success in that kind of environment is to enlist help from fitness-minded co-workers who want to do the 3-1-2-1 Diet too. Volunteer to bring nutritious foods to meetings, or ask the person in charge of the meeting to provide healthy fare like fresh fruit, yogurt, and whole-grain foods.

The best way to control overeating at work is to plan ahead. Pack your own healthy 3-1-2-1 Diet lunch and snacks. Stash a few small packets of almonds in your desk drawer and grab a piece of fruit instead of a candy bar when your energy nose-dives in the afternoon.

After work, it's fun to join your colleagues for happy hour, with drinks and appetizers. But watch yourself. It's easy to drink too much alcohol after a long, stressful day, or indulge in the most fattening appetizers. I suggest starting out with some carbonated water, and maybe an alcoholic drink or two after that (sip them; don't chug them). Take charge when it's time to order appetizers, and lobby for the healthiest choices, like shrimp cocktail, veggies and hummus, or grilled chicken tenders.

## DEALING WITH THE UNEXPECTED

There will be times when impromptu invitations hit: Someone drops by or sticks his head in your office door and suggests ordering a pizza or having dinner after a movie. It's a good idea to take a few moments to think clearly about how to handle the situation. You may decide to join in, especially if it's your cheat day, or go ahead with the invitation, intentionally making good food choices. If you've already eaten, perhaps you can suggest another time or say you'll eat a tiny amount. The key here is still planning, even if you have to do it on the fly.

## THE LIFE CRISIS

As someone like me knows: Life is not pain-free. There are going to be crises in your life: job loss, breakups and divorce, bankruptcy, a serious illness, or loss of a loved one. When that crisis hits—and it will—you have to be extra-careful about your health because you'll want to mask the pain, perhaps by bingeing, drinking too much alcohol, taking drugs, or engaging in other destructive behavior. If you go there, well, sometimes it's tough to turn back.

When you've got relatively smooth sailing in life, it's easier to find your way to the treadmill or the produce section for healthy, fresh food. But when you come under fire or are immersed in a crisis, it's just as easy to topple down the hill, one slippery fat gram at a time. Once the crisis has passed, you get a look at yourself in the mirror, and uh-oh, all that food you binged on is superglued to your hips, rear, and tummy. Not being able to deal constructively with crisis is the stuff yo-yo diets are made of. And I don't want you to yo-yo anymore; I want this program to be a lifestyle change for you.

Your best strategy for staying in control of yourself when the inevitable crisis hits is to have a plan. Take the positives you've learned and adapted so far from following the 3-1-2-1 Diet and exercise program, and have them in your psychological hip pocket for the stressful times. For example, if you've discovered that exercise has helped you cope with stress, then expand that experience by learning activities like yoga or tai chi (terrific substitutes for overeating in times of crisis) and add them to your crisis-management plan. Or perhaps you'll want to learn various relaxation techniques like massage or meditation because they are such effective antidotes to stress.

Commit ahead of any crisis that no matter what happens in your life, you will practice good self-care. Your body becomes more resilient to the negative effects of stress if you eat healthfully, take time to exercise, get adequate sleep, laugh and enjoy life, and stop trying to escape your problems with food. Healthy activities leave you feeling in better control of your life. Let's face it: No one feels in control when they're on their third package of cookies during a stressful situation. But when you eat well, get some physical activity, and practice other good habits, you naturally feel more empowered to manage your crisis.

Finally, strengthen your problem-solving skills. I hate to admit it, but a lot of crises that come our way are of our own making, and they usually don't resolve on their own. You have to take some sort of action. Let's say you're in debt over your head, and the situation is driving you to eat. Solving the problem might involve working with a financial counselor to set up a debt repayment plan, or changing your personal spending behaviors to avoid debt in the future. Some stressful aspects of our lives can be eliminated, reduced, or altered in a way that lessens their impact. Whatever the problem, there is always a solution. Try to isolate exactly what is making you feel stressed. Brainstorm all possible solutions and options without judgment, then narrow solutions down to the most workable and the most effective. Act on them, and evaluate how they worked.

Some people say that in crisis there is opportunity. And I think that is something to take seriously even if all you can see is the bad stuff. I would say that perhaps this means it's time to take charge and to live less reactively. When bad stuff hits, we come face-to-face with problems we've been hiding from. Do you need to get out of debt, mend fences with someone, take better care of your health, or something else? Face it, own up to it, solve it—and get on with your life.

I'm not preaching here (okay, maybe I am a little bit), but I think it's important to not focus on the woe-is-me part of it but rather to focus on how you're going to come out stronger, smarter, and wiser on account of going through it. Everything, no matter how dark it might seem at the time, comes together for good.

# 12 If You're Thinking *NO*, Add a *W*!

 $\text{C}$ all this chapter a pep talk, a coaching session, or just a one-on-one with you and me, but what I want is to close our time together with some thoughts about the mind-set we need to succeed in our fitness endeavors. I can't be with you every single day to help you reach your goal, but I can leave you with some advice that I'd like you to own and internalize.

Don't worry. I'm not going to tell you to "just think positive." That's like telling someone who's overweight to "just be skinny." To stay the course, to get in shape, and to stay fit, you've got to really want it. That's something I call "heart-core motivation." I can't give you that, but I can encourage you in that direction. So as we go through this final chapter together, hold in your heart all the reasons you have for getting and staying healthy and fit.

If there's one thing I've learned through my work on *The Biggest Loser*, it's that getting healthy and losing weight is as much of a mental battle as it is a physical one. As a trainer, I realize that there is more weight on the mind of an overweight person than on their body. My goal—my constant job—is to remind each person that they are good enough to take care of themselves and get in shape. If and when they realize that and put it into practice, then I've done my job. Let me start out by saying, if you ever think, "No, this isn't working in my life," add a *W*, and know you change things *NOW*.

## THE HABITS OF HEALTH

Aside from the physical challenges that *The Biggest Loser* contestants face on a weekly basis, psychological and emotional issues can have a huge impact on health, fitness, and the ability to push your body to the limit in order to effect positive change. Psychological factors are as much of a challenge to us trainers as they are to the contestants who are struggling with them, and it's tough to battle someone else's mind. I get frustrated sometimes, and I yell at my team because I don't have a lot of time to waste, but while doing that, I take a breath and encourage them that there's nothing they cannot do! Sometimes you have to destroy in order to rebuild.

Here's an analogy: Suppose you want to build a new house on a little plot of land. The problem is, there's a dilapidated old barn sitting right on the spot where you want to build your house. You've got to tear down that old barn first, right? Yes, and as people who want to look better, feel better, and live longer, we have to get rid of the old, bad habits standing in our way.

Habits are funny creatures. They often rule our lives, and we don't even realize we've developed them, whether they are good or bad. Habits are formed through our thoughts and our choices, and they take on lives of their own. If you can change your thoughts, you can change your choices, and ultimately your habits.

A really powerful and often limiting habit is how we deal with our emotions. Emotions—either positive or negative—can drive us toward food for comfort or escape. We have a saying on the show that tears are heavier than the pounds. It's so true. When we're dealing with loneliness, anxiety, boredom, depression—even joy—many of us reach for food. You want to eat because you equate food with comfort. Eating feels good, so most people (fat and thin alike) end up habitually using food as a ready source of emotional release or a way to ease stress and anxiety.

I remember Bonnie, an older lady who was a contestant on the *Biggest Loser*. She suffered from emotional overeating. Food comforted her. She had a knee injury, too, so she sat on the couch a lot, feeling sorry for herself. I eventually trained her, and I took a gentle but tough approach with her. I related to her pain. I told her I understood what she had been going through because I had once been sidelined by an injury. But I told her she had options that would get her moving again. One of those options was doing pool exercises. No one had brought that to her attention before. She became excited about her training again. She just needed an encouraging shove in the right direction and a positive tool she could use. No matter how low you go, there are always options to rise above that pain.

Of course, the unfortunate bottom line of emotional eating is weight gain, which in turn causes many people to feel worse about themselves, motivating still more mood-triggered eating and additional weight gain. Once you learn to strategize more dependable ways to deal with eating-related emotions, the sooner you can construct a departing point for emotional eating, leave it behind, and move forward beyond it.

I'll admit that emotional overeating does make you feel better, but not for long. For instance, researchers discovered that eating chocolate boosts a person's mood for only 3 minutes. Is emotional overeating worth it? No way. Instead of turning to food for comfort, I'd rather see you start building an arsenal of positive coping mechanisms that do last. My go-to activities in times of stress are working out, reading, writing, and meditating. Have tools like those available when you're in emotional pain. Here are some others to consider:

- Introduce new, enjoyable, or stimulating activities into your daily schedule.
- Keep yourself busy and have a more structured schedule to prevent boredom. Write letters, dig in the garden, organize items in your house, or do some volunteer work. Figure out how to use your free time for fun.
- Explore new hobbies or interests to deal with boredom. Are there activities you've always wanted to do but have never gotten around to doing? Follow through and make plans to do so.
- Redirect your activity and do something different. For example, rather than stay home by yourself and risk feeling lonely, call a friend and invite him or her out to a movie or other activity, or simply call a friend and talk on the phone.
- Learn to relax through meditation or other forms of relaxation as a component of developing a healthy lifestyle. The practice of meditation is a positive alternative to overeating or bingeing.
- Come to grips directly with whatever is troubling you. For example, if it's a problem with a relationship, talk it out. If it's your job, schedule a meeting with your boss to iron things out. In cases where you can't confront someone, at least do some physical activity. It is a great way to instantly feel better and slough off stress.
- Move. Exercise is a great cure for depression. Numerous studies have shown that physical activity can ease mild forms of depression. I know that when I'm in pain, I train!

- Get involved in meaningful experiences that relate to your religious beliefs, appeal to your creative talents, or help other people. Activities such as volunteering or using your talents bring meaning to your life, taking you outside yourself while focusing on others. Doing something for someone else lifts your spirits and lessens your own stress.

- See a person you like in the mirror each morning. This might be hard initially. You must first decide that you are worthwhile and valuable, because you are. There is only one of you, and you have special gifts and a purpose to offer the world. Affirm this repeatedly.

- If you suffer from ongoing depression—feelings of worthlessness, irritability, low energy, or a lack of pleasure in things you normally enjoy—consult a physician or mental health professional. Depression must be taken seriously. If we can locate the source of our pain, it's at that moment we face our demons, and then positive change begins.

## DON'T "CAN'T" YOURSELF

Another thought habit that will give you trouble is believing that you can't do something—like sticking to the diet or exercise routine. I tell clients and contestants all the time to curse at me, cuss me out, or scream; just don't "can't" me. That is my number one rule. If you tell me, "I can't do this," then we have some major issues, because you're just hurting yourself in the end. It's this kind of thinking that can make you feel like a failure and weaken your resolve even more.

People will get on the treadmill and limit themselves to a certain intensity, for example, and believe they cannot break through that barrier. Or they'll do an exercise routine only halfheartedly because they believe that's all their body is capable of. I'll ask them, and not gently: "Why are you letting this machine or routine control you? Aren't you sick and tired of other things controlling you?" So as they are doing that treadmill or routine, I sing those questions into them and place those issues on their heart. Those questions stick. They express the voice of reason within their mind of doubt.

One of my favorite sayings is "Tell your mind to get out of your body's way." This is a matter of saying positive, accurate things to yourself at your weakest hour so that you don't talk yourself out of the possible. Once people get this, I back off and they start owning their capacity to push themselves. And before long, they realize they can succeed.

Take John from season 12, for example. He had been training with Bob Harper, when he got reassigned to me. John didn't like the switch, so he told me he couldn't do this, or he wouldn't do that. I decided to prove him wrong.

John was on the treadmill, and I kept talking to him about his family, his wife, and his little boy. At the same time, I kept spiking the treadmill speed up until it finally got to 9.5 (that's high speed, folks!). Finally, I said to John, "Do you realize that you're running at nine and a half miles per hour?"

"Oh my God, I can't believe it," he said. John wanted to celebrate right there on the spot. He jumped off the treadmill and gave me the biggest hug possible. "Had you not been here, I would not have done that, but now I see that I can."

It's moments like those that make me want to celebrate too.

My point, though, is that you can do anything you put your mind to, whether in overcoming a specific challenge or reaching an important life goal. You've got to think big, push yourself, and go for it. Even I have to relearn that lesson from time to time.

I once participated in a television show called *Stars and Stripes*, in which military ops guys were paired with celebrities. The show aired on NBC during the Olympics. There were some tough physical challenges. I had to shoot live ammunition from machine guns and handguns. I had to lob grenades. I had to practice rescue missions. I even had to jump out of a helicopter in full gear into the water. And I'm not a great swimmer. Problem was, I had a broken foot so it was difficult for me to do all this. And I almost drowned! As it turned out, I was the first person eliminated from the competition.

Someone asked me, "Why did you do it?"

I said, "I may not be good at everything, but I am good at trying, and I like to challenge myself. It's a mind-set I've developed over many years."

The good news is that you can develop a fitness mind-set too. If the way you think about your body or your health is negative and causing you to fail, you can challenge and change it. What we focus on, we become. Get rid of thoughts that are standing in your way and limiting you. With the right fitness mind-set, you can begin to change your health trajectory.

Specifically, visualize what's possible for you: a new, healthy, in-shape, and energetic future for yourself. Imagine how wonderful you will feel and look. Go to work on that vision, and practice seeing your new self in your mind's eye. What you consciously think about, you will subconsciously move toward. Every thought has the power to defeat your goals or transform your life into everything you want it to be. It's your choice.

When my life transformed to success and happiness after growing up in an abusive home, it wasn't because I suddenly got luckier. I went from getting beaten down, physically and mentally, to building a successful fitness business because I developed the right mind-set and strength of spirit, as if my life depended on it...which it clearly did. My childhood lessons programmed me to draw from the truths I knew in order to deal with the future I did not know. I learned that in seemingly impossible situations there is a way to become unshakable through setbacks.

If you want massive transformation in your life, you must create a can-do mind-set that is conditioned and programmed to succeed no matter what. I remember one *Biggest Loser* episode in which the contestants participated in a 5K run as one of their challenges. Many of them would never have dreamed that they could ever complete a 5K run, but I think all of the contestants amazed themselves and caught a glimpse of their tremendous potential.

For any of you readers out there who are worried that you'll never be able to complete a 5K, I have some advice. If you practice a walk or jog every day, you will eventually be able to run effortlessly. Start simple, keep moving however you can, and build up your strength and skills. Put in the time to improve and your body will surprise you. There's no better feeling in the world than starting out thinking you can't do something, and you do it anyway.

We have choices in life; we all do. We can choose to believe in ourselves or doubt ourselves, but we have that choice. What if I said to you: There is nothing you can't do? *Well, I can't jump out of a plane and I can't be a billionaire and I can't—* What if you could? Would you do everything it takes to get to that space? There is nothing you can't do—even if that little voice inside you says you can't. Guess what? You control that voice too. It is entirely up to you.

Great health and fitness are never accidents. You can't focus on creating fitness and health, then accidentally create poor fitness and an out-of-shape body. Fitness is the result of a determined, disciplined approach to life. Having the right mind-set is your personal GPS to guide you to your goals.

You've got to own the 3-1-2-1 Diet as your lifestyle, along with exercising. Once these things are in place as brand-new habits, you'll get a different result than you have before. You'll reach your goal weight. You'll stay at that weight. You'll enjoy your favorite foods. You'll waste no calories on foods you don't like. Your lifestyle will include every kind of meat, restaurant food, wine, recipe, and even dessert you can think of, as long as you eat them in moderation. You'll deny yourself nothing. This diet reprograms your habits so that your calories come out right, and the whole program becomes habitual and easy to maintain for life.

I don't want to be known as the trainer who has the most winners. I want to be known as the trainer who taught the most people to keep weight off. I want to be that guy. If I can do that—I have done my job. But that job isn't to stick to someone for the rest of their life; my job is to make them—and you—independent. Your transformation always begins with you. You can't wait for someone to push you along, because the drive and intention must come from you.

Choose thoughts and actions that build you up, not tear you down. Believe you can achieve. Know that you are worth it and that you are a beautiful person on the inside and outside. Stay focused on what you would have in your life. Believe that you can create and make your goals happen, make your life change, and live the life you've always wanted. Just around the corner of your life are things you've never dreamed possible.

# APPENDIX

# My Training Log

Your Training Log is easy to fill out. Mostly, you simply check off each item that you complete successfully, and fill in the amount of time you devote to cardio or your fun activity. The beauty of this type of training log is that after you fill it out, look at your check marks, and you'll see all that you've accomplished each day. The log helps keep you accountable—and inspired. Instead of check marks, you can use gold stars or other motivating stickers.

| DAY 1. Date: | |
|---|---|
| *First Cardio Timed Sequence* | *Duration in Minutes (strive for 10 minutes)* |
| ❏  March in place | |
| ❏  Run/jog in place | |
| ❏  Treadmill | |
| *Lower-Body Timed Sequence: 10 Minutes of Strength Training* | |
| ❏  Squats or Resistance Band Squats for 2 minutes | |
| ❏  Forward Lunge or Resistance Band Lunge for 2 minutes | |
| ❏  Backward Lunge for 2 minutes | |
| ❏  Dead Lifts for 2 minutes | |
| ❏  Sumo Squats for 1 minute | |
| ❏  Hamstring Lifts for 1 minute | |

*continued*

| DAY 1 *continued* |
|---|

| Second Cardio Timed Sequence | Duration in Minutes (strive for 8 minutes) |
|---|---|
| ❏ Jump rope<br>❏ Run up and down stairs<br>❏ Home cardio equipment | |

| Upper-Body Large-Muscle Timed Sequence: 8 Minutes of Strength Training |
|---|
| ❏ Alternate Push-ups and Planks for 2 minutes |
| ❏ Chest Butterfly Press on Mat or Butterfly Press with a Resistance Band for 2 minutes |
| ❏ Dumbbell Chest Press for 2 minutes |
| ❏ Dumbbell Pullover for 1 minute |
| ❏ Dumbbell Rows or Resistance Band Rows for 1 minute |

| Third Cardio Timed Sequence | Duration in Minutes (strive for 6 minutes) |
|---|---|
| ❏ Jump rope<br>❏ Run up and down stairs<br>❏ Home cardio equipment | |

| Upper-Body Small-Muscle Timed Sequence: 6 Minutes of Strength Training |
|---|
| ❏ Shoulder Press for 1 minute |
| ❏ Side Laterals with a Resistance Band for 1 minute |
| ❏ Biceps Hammer Curls or Resistance Band Hammer Curls for 2 minutes |
| ❏ Triceps Kickbacks with Dumbbells or a Resistance Band for 2 minutes |

| DAY 2. Date: |
|---|

| First Cardio Timed Sequence | Duration in Minutes (strive for 10 minutes) |
|---|---|
| ❏ March in place<br>❏ Run/jog in place<br>❏ Treadmill | |

| *Lower-Body Timed Sequence: 10 Minutes of Strength Training* | |
| --- | --- |
| ❏  Squats or Resistance Band Squats for 2 minutes | |
| ❏  Forward Lunge or Resistance Band Lunge for 2 minutes | |
| ❏  Backward Lunge for 2 minutes | |
| ❏  Dead Lifts for 2 minutes | |
| ❏  Sumo Squats for 1 minute | |
| ❏  Hamstring Lifts for 1 minute | |
| *Second Cardio Timed Sequence* | *Duration in minutes (strive for 8 minutes)* |
| ❏  Jump rope<br>❏  Run up and down stairs<br>❏  Home cardio equipment | |
| *Upper-Body Large-Muscle Timed Sequence: 8 Minutes of Strength Training* | |
| ❏  Alternate Push-ups and Planks for 2 minutes | |
| ❏  Chest Butterfly Press on Mat or Butterfly Press with a Resistance Band for 2 minutes | |
| ❏  Dumbbell Chest Press for 2 minutes | |
| ❏  Dumbbell Pullover for 1 minute | |
| ❏  Dumbbell Rows or Resistance Band Rows for 1 minute | |
| *Third Cardio Timed Sequence* | *Duration in Minutes (strive for 6 minutes)* |
| ❏  Jump rope<br>❏  Run up and down stairs<br>❏  Home cardio equipment | |
| *Upper-Body Small-Muscle Timed Sequence: 6 Minutes of Strength Training* | |
| ❏  Shoulder Press for 1 minute | |
| ❏  Side Laterals with a Resistance Band for 1 minute | |
| ❏  Biceps Hammer Curls or Resistance Band Hammer Curls for 2 minutes | |
| ❏  Triceps Kickbacks with Dumbbells or a Resistance Band for 2 minutes | |

*continued*

| DAY 3. Date: | |
| --- | --- |
| *First Cardio Timed Sequence* | *Duration in Minutes (strive for 6 minutes)* |
| ❑  March in place<br>❑  Run/jog in place<br>❑  Treadmill | |
| *Lower-Body Timed Sequence: 6 Minutes of Strength Training* | |
| ❑  Squats or Resistance Band Squats for 2 minutes<br>❑  Forward Lunge or Resistance Band Lunge for 2 minutes<br>❑  Dead Lifts for 2 minutes | |
| *Second Cardio Timed Sequence* | *Duration in Minutes (strive for 8 minutes)* |
| ❑  Jump rope<br>❑  Run up and down stairs<br>❑  Home cardio equipment | |
| *Upper-Body Large-Muscle Timed Sequence: 8 Minutes of Strength Training* | |
| ❑  Alternate Push-ups and Planks for 1 minute<br>❑  Chest Butterfly Press on Mat or Butterfly Press with a Resistance Band for 2 minutes<br>❑  Dumbbell Chest Press for 2 minutes<br>❑  Dumbbell Pullover for 1 minute<br>❑  Dumbbell Rows or Resistance Band Rows for 2 minutes | |
| *Third Cardio Timed Sequence* | *Duration in Minutes (strive for 10 minutes)* |
| ❑  March in place<br>❑  Run/jog in place<br>❑  Treadmill | |
| *Upper-Body Small-Muscle Timed Sequence: 10 Minutes of Strength Training* | |
| ❑  Shoulder Press for 2 minutes<br>❑  Side Laterals with a Resistance Band for 2 minutes | |

- ❏ Biceps Hammer Curls or Resistance Band Hammer Curls for 2 minutes
- ❏ Triceps/Shoulder Lifts with a Resistance Band for 2 minutes
- ❏ Triceps Kickbacks with Dumbbells or a Resistance Band for 2 minutes

| DAY 4. Date: | |
|---|---|
| *First Cardio Timed Sequence* | *Duration in Minutes (strive for 6 minutes)* |
| ❏ March in place<br>❏ Run/jog in place<br>❏ Treadmill | |
| *Lower-Body Timed Sequence: 6 Minutes of Strength Training* | |
| ❏ Squats or Resistance Band Squats for 2 minutes | |
| ❏ Forward Lunge or Resistance Band Lunge for 2 minutes | |
| ❏ Dead Lifts for 2 minutes | |
| *Second Cardio Timed Sequence* | *Duration in Minutes (strive for 8 minutes)* |
| ❏ Jump rope<br>❏ Run up and down stairs<br>❏ Home cardio equipment | |
| *Upper-Body Large-Muscle Timed Sequence: 8 Minutes of Strength Training* | |
| ❏ Alternate Push-ups and Planks for 1 minute | |
| ❏ Chest Butterfly Press on Mat or Butterfly Press with a Resistance Band for 2 minutes | |
| ❏ Dumbbell Chest Press for 2 minutes | |
| ❏ Dumbbell Pullover for 1 minute | |
| ❏ Dumbbell Rows or Resistance Band Rows for 2 minutes | |

*continued*

| DAY 4. *continued* | |
|---|---|
| *Third Cardio Timed Sequence* | *Duration in Minutes (strive for 10 minutes)* |
| ❏ March in place<br>❏ Run/jog in place<br>❏ Treadmill | |
| *Upper-Body Small-Muscle Timed Sequence: 10 Minutes of Strength Training* | |
| ❏ Shoulder Press for 2 minutes | |
| ❏ Side Laterals with a Resistance Band for 2 minutes | |
| ❏ Biceps Hammer Curls or Resistance Band Hammer Curls for 2 minutes | |
| ❏ Triceps/Shoulder Lifts with a Resistance Band for 2 minutes | |
| ❏ Triceps Kickbacks with Dumbbells or a Resistance Band for 2 minutes | |

| Rest, DAY 5 |
|---|

| Cardio, DAY 6. Date: | |
|---|---|
| *Exercise* | *Time Spent (Duration) (strive for at least 60 minutes)* |
| | |

| Active Fun, DAY 7. Date: | |
|---|---|
| *Exercise* | *Time Spent (Duration) (strive for at least 60 minutes)* |
| | |

# REFERENCES

Ahmadi, N., Eshaghian, S., Huizenga, R., Sosnin, K., Ebrahimi, R., and Siegel, R. 2011. Effects of intense exercise and moderate caloric restriction on cardiovascular risk factors and inflammation. *American Journal of Medicine* 124:978–982.

Arciero, P.J., Ormsbee, M.J., Gentile, C.L., et al. 2013. Increased protein intake and meal frequency reduces abdominal fat during energy balance and energy deficit. *Obesity*, January 2.

Baer, D.J., Stote, K.S., Paul, D.R., et al. 2011. Whey protein but not soy protein supplementation alters body weight and composition in free-living overweight and obese adults. *Journal of Nutrition* 141:1489–1494.

Bermudez, O., and Gao, X. 2010. Greater consumption of sweetened beverages and added sugars is associated with obesity among U.S. young adults. *Annals of Nutrition and Metabolism* 57:211–218.

Bescós, R., Sureda, A., Tur, J.A., and Pons, A. 2012. The effect of nitric-oxide-related supplements on human performance. *Sports Medicine* 42:99–117.

Brennan, I.M., Luscombe-Marsh, N.D., Seimon, R.V., et al. 2012. Effects of fat, protein, and carbohydrate and protein load on appetite, plasma cholecystokinin, peptide YY, and ghrelin, and energy intake in lean and obese men. *American Journal of Physiology, Gastrointestinal and Liver Physiology* 303:G129–140.

Burke, L.E., Wang, J., and Sevick, M.A. 2011. Self-monitoring in weight loss: a systematic review of the literature. *Journal of the American Dietetic Association* 111:92–102.

Chen, S.C., Lin, Y.H., Huang, H.P., et al. 2012. Effect of conjugated linoleic acid supplementation on weight loss and body fat composition in a Chinese population. *Nutrition* 28:559–565.

Clare, B.A., Conroy, R.S., and Spelman, K. 2009. The diuretic effect in human subjects of an extract of Taraxacum officinale folium over a single day. *Journal of Alternative and Complementary Medicine* 15:929–934.

Coker, R.H., Miller, S., and Schutzler, S. 2012. Whey protein and essential amino acids promote the reduction of adipose tissue and increased muscle protein synthesis during caloric restriction-induced weight loss in elderly, obese individuals. *Nutrition Journal* 11:105.

Di Pasquale, M. 1997. *Amino Acids and Proteins for the Athlete: The Anabolic Edge.* New York: CRC Press.

Forbes, G.B., et al. 1989. Hormonal response to overfeeding. *American Journal of Clinical Nutrition* 49:608–611.

Gaullier, J.M., Halse, J., Høivik, H.O., et al. 2007. Six months supplementation with conjugated linoleic acid induces regional-specific fat mass decreases in overweight and obese. *British Journal of Nutrition* 97:550–560.

Gregersen, N.T., Belza, A., Jensen, M.G., et al. 2012. Acute effects of mustard, horseradish, black pepper and ginger on energy expenditure, appetite, ad libitum energy intake and energy balance in human subjects. *British Journal of Nutrition* 5:1–8.

Gualano, A.B., Bozza, T., Lopes De Campos, P., et al. 2011. Branched-chain amino acids supplementation enhances exercise capacity and lipid oxidation during endurance exercise after muscle glycogen depletion. *Journal of Sports Medicine and Physical Fitness* 51:82–88.

Hairston, K.G. et al. 2012. Lifestyle factors and 5-year abdominal fat accumulation in a minority cohort: the IRAS Family Study. *Obesity* 20: 421–427.

House, J.D., Neufeld, J., and Leson, G. 2010. Evaluating the quality of protein from hemp seed (Cannabis sativa L.) products through the use of the protein digestibility-corrected amino acid score method. *Journal of Agricultural and Food Chemistry* 58:11801–11807.

Ibrügger, S., Kristensen, M., Mikkelsen, M.S., and Astrup, A. 2012. Flaxseed dietary fiber supplements for suppression of appetite and food intake. *Appetite* 58:490–495.

Illian, T.G., Casey, J.C., and Bishop, P.A. 2011. Omega 3 chia seed loading as a means of carbohydrate loading. *Journal of Strength and Conditioning Research* 25:61–65.

Jebb, S.A., et al. 1996. Changes in macronutrient balance during over- and underfeeding assessed by 12-day continuous whole-body calorimetry. *American Journal of Clinical Nutrition* 64:259–266.

Johnston, C.S., Day, C.S., and Swan, P.D. 2002. Postprandial thermogenesis is increased 100% on a high-protein, low-fat diet versus a high-carbohydrate, low-fat diet in healthy, young women. *Journal of the American College of Nutrition* 21:55–61.

Johnston, C.S., Steplewska, I., Long, C.A., et al. 2010. Examination of the antiglycemic properties of vinegar in healthy adults. *Annals of Nutrition and Metabolism* 56:74–79.

Kalman, D.S., Feldman, S., et al. 2012. Comparison of coconut water and a carbohydrate-electrolyte sport drink on measures of hydration and physical performance in exercise-trained men. *Journal of the International Society of Sports Nutrition* 9:1.

Kerksick, C., Harvey, T., Stout, J., et al. 2008. International Society of Sports Nutrition position stand: nutrient timing. *International Society of Sports Nutrition* 5:17.

Larson-Meyer, D.E., Willis, K.S., and Willis, L.M. 2010. Effect of honey versus sucrose on appetite, appetite-regulating hormones, and postmeal thermogenesis. *Journal of the American College of Nutrition* 29:482–493.

Mansour, M.S., Ni, Y.M., Roberts, A.L., et al. 2012. Ginger consumption enhances the thermic effect of food and promotes feelings of satiety without affecting metabolic and hormonal parameters in overweight men: a pilot study. *Metabolism* 61:1347–1352.

Maughan, R.J., et al. 1997. Diet composition and the performance of high-intensity exercise. *Journal of Sport Science* 15:265–275.

Munro, I.A., and Garg, M.L. 2013. Prior supplementation with long chain omega-3 polyunsaturated fatty acids promotes weight loss in obese adults: a double-blinded randomised controlled trial. *Food & Function* 4:650–658.

Nackers, L.M., et al. 2010. The association between rate of initial weight loss and long-term success in obesity treatment: does slow and steady win the race? *International Journal of Behavioral Medicine* 17:161–167.

Newby, P.K., Muller, D., Hallfrisch, J., et al. 2003. Dietary patterns and changes in body mass index and waist circumference in adults. *American Journal of Clinical Nutrition* 77:1417–1425.

Ostman, E., Granfeldt, Y., Persson, L., and Björck, I. 2005. Vinegar supplementation lowers glucose and insulin responses and increases satiety after a bread meal in healthy subjects. *European Journal of Clinical Nutrition* 59:983–988.

Ostojic, S.M. 2006. Yohimbine: the effects on body composition and exercise performance in soccer players. *Research in Sports and Medicine* 14:289–299.

Paoli, A., Pacelli, F., Bargossi, A.M., et al. 2010. Effects of three distinct protocols of fitness training on body composition, strength and blood lactate. *Journal of Sports Medicine and Physical Fitness* 50:43–51.

Prasad, K. 2009. Flaxseed and cardiovascular health. *Journal of Cardiovascular Pharmacology* 54:369–377.

Rock, C.L., Emond, J.A., and Flatt, S.W. 2012. Weight loss is associated with increased serum 25-hydroxyvitamin D in overweight or obese women. *Obesity* 20:2296–2301.

Rothwell, J., et al. 1985. Hormonal and metabolic responses to fasting and refeeding. *International Journal of Obesity* 9(Suppl 2): 49–54.

Roy, H.J., et al. 1998. Substrate oxidation and energy expenditure in athletes and nonathletes consuming isoenergetic high- and low-fat diets. *American Journal of Clinical Nutrition* 67:405–411.

Saris, W.H. 1995. Effects of energy restriction and exercise on the sympathetic nervous system. *International Journal of Obesity and Related Metabolic Disorders* 19(Suppl 7): S17S23.

Sharp, C.P., and Pearson, D.R. 2010. Amino acid supplements and recovery from high-intensity resistance training. *Journal of Strength Conditioning and Research* 24:1125–1130.

Stanhope, K.L., and Havel, P.J. 2008. Fructose consumption: potential mechanisms for its effects to increase visceral adiposity and induce dyslipidemia and insulin resistance. *Current Opinion in Lipidology* 19:16–24.

Stanhope, K.L., Schwarz, J.M., and Keim, N.L. 2009. Consuming fructose-sweetened, not glucose-sweetened, beverages increases visceral adiposity and lipids and decreases insulin sensitivity in overweight/obese humans. *Journal of Clinical Investigation* 119: 1322–1334.

Tan, S.T., Tapsell, L., Batterham, M., and Charlton, K. 2008. Defining the functional properties of dietary protein and protein-rich foods in human energy expenditure. *Nutrition & Dietetics* 65 (Suppl. 3): S66–S70.

Ulbricht, C., Chao, W., Nummy, K., et al. 2009. Chia (Salvia hispanica): a systematic review by the natural standard research collaboration. *Reviews on Recent Clinical Trials* 4:168–174.

Whigham, L.D., Watras, A.C., and Schoeller, D.A. 2007. Efficacy of conjugated linoleic acid for reducing fat mass: a meta-analysis in humans. *American Journal of Clinical Nutrition* 85:1203–1211.

Whiting, S., Derbyshire, E., and Tiwari, B.K. 2012. Capsaicinoids and capsinoids. A potential role for weight management? A systematic review of the evidence. *Appetite* 59: 341–348.

Wu, H., Pan, A., Yu, Z., et al. 2010. Lifestyle counseling and supplementation with flaxseed or walnuts influence the management of metabolic syndrome. *Journal of Nutrition* 140:1937–1942.

# INDEX

# ABOUT THE AUTHOR

Fitness expert and television star Dolvett Quince has quickly risen through the ranks as one of America's favorite trainers. He has completed several seasons on the hit NBC show *The Biggest Loser*, and his passion, regimen, and dramatic transformational results have made him one of the most in-demand fitness specialists in the country.

Dolvett moved from Connecticut to Atlanta to pursue his passion for fitness by becoming one of the most sought-after trainers in Atlanta. In 2004, he opened Body Sculptor, a private personal training studio with a commitment to "changing lives one rep at a time." His business had a solid following, but it wasn't until a local radio personality started talking about it on his show that Dolvett and his business really took off. He then widened his business to training other trainers, which then led to him training celebrities such as actors Angela Bassett, Boris Kodjoe, and Nicole Ari Parker, Baltimore Ravens tight end Daniel Wilcox, singer-songwriter Jojo, and world pop sensation Justin Bieber.

Within the studio, Dolvett created Pure Energy a high-intensity circuit-training class with a live DJ, which was voted Best Workout in the Southeast. The popularity of Dolvett's fitness methods inspired the launch of his own DVD, *Me and My Chair: The No Excuses Workout*, a low-impact, high-intensity 30-minute workout system that helps users tone up and slim down while using only a household chair.

Soon after, Dolvett was cast on *The Biggest Loser,* and during his first two seasons, he guided his team to two consecutive wins. He also appeared in the NBC series *Stars Earn Stripes* and guest starred on the first season of the new BET series *The Real Husbands of Hollywood*.

Dolvett is very passionate about giving back and helping others. He is an active supporter of nonprofit organizations such as Children's Healthcare of Atlanta, the American Heart Association, and Got Your 6, which helps veterans transition into civilian life.

Dolvett currently splits his time between Los Angeles and Atlanta and enjoys time with his son, Isiah.